CW00838707

My dearest Julie,

Enjoy my love,

Kelly xx.

HELP!
I can't see my
foo foo...

Diary of a first time pregnancy! A day to day
journey into a mother's life, her fears and her foo

Kelly O'Brien M.D (Mother Diva)

authorHOUSE®

AuthorHouse™
1663 Liberty Drive, Suite 200
Bloomington, IN 47403
www.authorhouse.com
Phone: 1-800-839-8640

©2008 Kelly O'Brien M.D (Mother Diva). All rights reserved.

No part of this book may be reproduced, stored in a retrieval system, or transmitted by any means without the written permission of the author.

First published by AuthorHouse   11/5/2008

Printed in the United States of America
Bloomington, Indiana

This book is printed on acid-free paper.

ISBN: 978-1-4259-6591-4 (sc)

Contents

Chapter 8

Chapter 9

Chapter 10

Intro...

My name is Kelly O'Brien. I am a mother, entertainer and writer.

I am not famous *(yet)* and this is my first book.

I am not a midwife or a doctor. I'm not a nutritionist nor do I work for the NHS. I am not an obstetrician or a gynaecologist. I am not a paediatrician or a biologist.

I have no expertise in writing this book other than having been pregnant, given birth and become a mother.

I have spread my legs and felt a watermelon sized baby come out of my vagina. My foo foo has been cut and stitched. I've had cracked nipples, haemorrhoids, aching feet, crying fits, stretch marks, a fat ass, an un-waxed bikini line for nine months and I've massaged my own asshole.

As far as I'm concerned any woman who has been through even half of this has the expertise to write whatever she damn wants.

Firstly however, I need to tell you a bit about myself, otherwise you might just think I'm a wanker!!

I was born in a small town in South Australia called McLaren Vale, to a 6 ft father and a 4 ft 10 inch mother, so I guess genetics saw to it that I would not grow very tall; *I am just 5 ft*. However, what I lacked in height I made up for in personality, and from a young age became an amateur comedienne and entertainer. I was also lucky enough to possess charisma, wit, and more front than K-Mart.

Being born with a great voice, my life plan was obviously well thought out by God. *(I was also fortunate enough to be a teenager right in the middle of the Karaoke Revolution.)* Therefore, it was inevitable that I HAD to be a singer. If I wasn't, I would have had to join the circus.

The problem was, I had absolutely NO IDEA how I would become a professional singer...

So I guessed.

I made it up as I went along.

And taught myself everything I know.

Since then I have been singing professionally for 14 years.

I have worked in jazz bands, blues bands, rock bands, piano bars, cabaret shows, and theatre restaurants. I've travelled with production companies to Thailand, Japan, Papua New Guinea, Taiwan, New Zealand, Germany and the UK. I've appeared in TV commercials, film clips, hosted breakfast shows, and had my own single reach number four in the Polish dance charts!!!

I've been Ginger Spice, Snow White, Minnie Mouse, Dolly Parton, Diana Ross, and a starfish. I was a finalist in TV's 'Popstars'.

I have met and worked with Drew Barrymore, Bruce Willis, Adam Sandler, Geena Davis, Tom Arnold, Kylie Minogue, and pressed Billy Zane's hands into concrete. I have hung out with Nicole Kidman and Tom Cruises kids, peed my pants while singing for Queen, danced half naked in front of Ewan McGregor and sung on Russell Crowe's ranch for two days.

I have spent the last 10 years expecting to get famous at any time.

Definitely not expecting a baby!

I never actually thought I wanted to have children *(well, not until about 2025 anyway)*. However, I got knocked up by new husband and by some wild decision, we decided to go for it.

I never in my wildest dreams thought I would be a mother at 28.

I was supposed to be fucking famous.

Realising I was going to have a baby scared the absolute shit out of me. I kept thinking I was making a terrible mistake, that I wasn't ready to become a mother. I didn't want my life to change. I thought I would have to throw away my dreams and my career. *(I also thought being a mother meant I had to put my hair up in a bun, wear an apron and never say the word 'fuck'.)*

I realised later however, that a mother can be whoever you want her to be. There are no rules.

Being an entertainer was amazing but it also made me completely self-obsessed. I was egocentric, self-centred and a complete show off, totally focussed on being a star. Becoming a mother changed that. *(Well, I'm still going to be a star, but now I have saggier tits.)* It slowed me down and showed me what is truly important in life.

It made me into a better person.

Pregnancy really is such a selfless act, and what a wonderful journey. I don't think I could experience such a unique and amazing transformation again *(unless I have a sex change operation or something?)*

I really got to know myself, and decided what kind of person I really wanted to be. Being a mum is better than performing to 50,000 people. It's better than taking drugs and even better than singing in a bikini at the Mardi Gras.

It's the best thing that I have ever done with my life.

What you are about to read is my diary. I've been writing in it since I was 13 years old but have decided to share the 12 months with you! I wrote almost every day of my pregnancy and my story is full of tears, laughter, courage, sadness and ecstasy. By the end of it, I experienced a part of myself I'd never known… including a very sore vag!

So sit back relax and enjoy my journey, along with your own.

N.B. The following words are used to describe the female vagina during the course of this book- Minge, Foo Foo, Punaani, Vag, Flaps, Vagina, Nooni, Moo Moo, Minnie and Fanny.

Kelly xxx

'In loving Memory of Martin Boothe'

Chapter 1

Petrified and Unqualified

"A period is the beginning of a life long sentence."
Cathy Crimmins

7 October 2002

Today I've found out that I am pregnant. I just cannot believe it!

I don't want to have a baby. I didn't want to get pregnant, but I am, oh my God. Fuck... I am in complete shock. I'm not ready for this. I'm only 27. I have a fantastic career and I look damn good; I don't want to get a big tummy and stretch marks.

I am supposed to be a big star.

PREGNANT, oh my God. Pregnant! *(I have to keep repeating it so it sinks in.)* This is not in my life plan; I mean how can I be pregnant? Now? Just when my life feels absolutely perfect? Holy shit. How did this happen? *(Um, yeah...I wonder?)*

It must have been all the sex I've been having with the new love of my life. His name is JC *(yes, as in Van Damme.)*

Anyway, we fell in love five months ago.

After two months I knew I wanted to marry him.

And after one week, I knew this was the kind of sex that a young woman could not live without; it was great, so of course there was plenty of it

So, that's HOW I got pregnant, but WHEN did it happen? Could have been anywhere between April and October *(though I doubt it would have been April since I would be 6 months pregnant by now)*. But WHY it's happened, I don't know.

I've never been pregnant before. This is quite amazing, considering I was a slut during my early twenties. But why has this happened now? I cannot believe it!

Pregnant now, when I have just moved from my home in Australia to Germany to star in the musical Starlight Express.

Pregnant now, when I have spent over £8,000 on plastic surgery in the past five years to look my damn best.

Pregnant now, when I have plans to become a major Superstar!

Pregnant now, when I paid good money for that fucking diaphragm, and it didn't even work.

Pregnant? Now?

How can it be?

I have always been so focused on becoming the most fabulously successful person anyone has ever met. I am talented and God already has a plan for me, a baby is just not in those plans!

My life was in those plans.

8 October

It all started a few days ago.

I had a meeting with the Company Manager of the show at the theatre. Firstly however, let me tell you a bit about my job at 'Starlight Express'.

For starters it's on roller skates. We are trains, and I play one of the lead roles. *(I am the Dining Car.)* Oh….. and it's in German.

Anyway, I was going in to talk about extending my contract with the show for another year, when on my way home I decided to randomly pick up a pregnancy test from the chemist because I had not seen any trace of my period for almost two months.

N.B. My periods have been completely irregular for the last ten years and usually come every six to eight weeks, so I was not too concerned that one was once again delayed.

It was just a normal Wednesday afternoon.

I had taken pregnancy tests before *(many many times)* and they had always turned out to be negative, so you can imagine how shocked I was when two little windows came up positive.

I was silent.

I stopped breathing.

I felt like I was in a dream.

Was this right? Surely not. I couldn't be pregnant…

But I was. And I knew it.

FUUUUUUUCCCCKKKK!

The first thing I did was cry. Tears of confusion, tears of amazement, tears of how the hell did this happen? And oddly enough… tears of joy.

I told JC straight away. *(JC is my abbreviation for Jean-Claude NOT Jesus Christ.)* He didn't seem to be as shocked as I was. He was actually more concerned about his overwhelmed and distraught girlfriend; however, I could see the sparkle in his eye, and I knew straight away that he wanted to keep the baby.

Firstly though, I needed confirmation. I needed to be extra sure. I needed to know whether my tears were justified, I needed to know that this little stupid pregnancy test was the real deal.

I went straight to the gynaecologist *(who was closed.)* So instead I went back to the chemist and picked up two more - top of the range, more expensive, more accurate than a lie detector - pregnancy tests. I quickly walked home, went into the toilet, piddled on the stick, piddled on the stick again; waited, waited some more, and then started to cry again.

They were both positive.

I rang work straight away. I was supposed to be on stage in less than two hours, but do you think I could fucking roller skate and sing in German with a bun in the oven? No way. All I was thinking was; "I can't have a baby now."

Secretly though, I must admit that I was a tiny bit excited by this new challenge life was throwing at me.

I just didn't know whether I wanted to be throwing up for the next three months?

9 October

All I have been thinking about for the last 24 hours is babies, babies, babies.

Do I want one? Do I want to become a mummy? Do I want to be like ten zillion women out there? Let me tell you: there is <u>nothing</u> glamorous whatsoever about being a mother.

Let me think… Mummy Dearest. The Mummy Returns. The Mamas and the Papas. Nope, none of those are cool.

I think I am still in shock and completely overwhelmed.

I have never been faced with making a choice like this before. I had always assumed that it would take a miracle for this to happen. Well I guess in a way it is a miracle, but am I ready for this?

I always thought that if I became pregnant by this stage of my life I could <u>never</u> have a child, but it feels different actually BEING pregnant.

I feel very calm and warm inside like chicken soup.

I feel excited and instantly important.

I feel petrified, yet at peace.

I feel like life has come knocking on the door and invited me to celebrate with the rest of the world.

I feel like I am being asked by Mother Nature to join in on a wonderfully unique experience.

I feel like I know a secret that no body else knows.

I feel like a woman. A real woman.

I'm sure JC really wants to keep the baby but he's not the one whose fanny is going to tear in half.

10 October.

Aaaaaaarrrgggghhhh.

My mind feels like it's about to melt. I still don't know what to do?

This decision about whether or not to keep this baby affects not only my life but JC's life too. He is only 19 years old for God's sake. I don't know of any man who would want a baby at 19. Fuck!

He really does want to have a baby with me though, and he is really excited at the prospect *(probably so I will cook and clean for him for the next 30 years).*

I cannot believe that I am more petrified than he is! He is so confident that we could have this baby. Oh my God, could we really do this? Are we bloody insane?

11 October.

Yes, we are insane.

We have decided to keep the baby. Holy shit.

I am scared/excited/petrified/anxious, however it just seems to feel right. I guess the decision was ultimately up to me because obviously it's my body that is going to go through pregnancy and childbirth. However, JC and I did have a long talk about everything and how wonderful it would be to have a child together. Where we are both headed career wise? Where we are financially? Where we will live? *(He is from England, and I am from Australia.)* Where would our child grow up? How would it affect our relationship as a couple? And would we ever find time to have sex again? The talk actually left me feeling great and confident, and quite excited about becoming a parent.

So we eventually made it into the office at work today to tell the Director and choreographer of our plans, and they actually seemed genuinely thrilled for us. I was really nervous beforehand, like a 12 year old girl summoned to the head master's office. However, they were both great and very supportive, although they insisted that I stop work immediately. They will obviously have to find a replacement for me asap. *(I felt quite uncomfortable about this.)* Needless to say they were very understanding and assured me that the miracle of life was more important than anything else in this world. *(Are these people for real or what?)*

12 October.

I went to a gynaecologist today. Her name is Mrs Zeidler. She is wonderful and speaks fantastic English. *(Always helpful when you're talking about your vag.)* I found out that I am actually six weeks pregnant. Wow. I had no idea. Anyway, she took some urine, blood, and gave me a tiny booklet, a pat on the back and a little picture of a tiny blob which is supposed to be the most amazing thing I will ever experience in my life. How weird.

I called my Mum and Dad in Australia today.

"Mum, guess what?" I said.

"You're gonna have a baby?" she replied.

"Oh my God, how did you know?"

"I just knew," she said. "Mother's intuition."

Jeez, she took all the fun out of it.

Then I spoke to Dad and he was thrilled, although I felt a bit guilty that he has never met JC and given his approval. *(Dads like to do that!)*

I also told my sisters Adele and Peta.

Peta said; "Oh…..Cool."

"Oh cool… Is that it?" I thought

"Aren't you surprised at all?" I asked. "Aren't you shocked? And think I'm insane?"

"No," Peta replied. "I was surprised when you told me you were a lesbian once, and I was surprised when you said you were going to get a boob job, but NO I can't say I'm surprised by this."

Adele on the other hand was extremely surprised; "Oh my goodness. Really? That is so wonderful, how amazing, that's so fantastic, congratulations, congratulations, you will be a fabulous mother, you must be so excited."

BINGO! See, that's what I'm talking about! That is exactly the kind of response you want to hear once you've made plans to become a parent and ruin your life; it's a big deal, and I won't let anyone convince me otherwise.

Adele has two children already with her husband Matt and they are expecting their third child in December. I am definitely not going to need any of those stupid pregnancy magazines with her only a phone call away. She is going to be a marvellous help to me in the next nine months; she is a wonderful mother.

13 October

I am feeling rather sick and have been sleeping all day.

While I slept, I actually dreamt of two names for the baby, Kitten and Velvet.

JC hates them both.

I also went into the gynaecologist's earlier and had about a hundred tests; it was so painfully boring *(except for the blood tests - they were just painful)*. They checked my weight, my blood pressure, my urine, my blood type, you name it, they did it. They even gave me a HIV test. *(Shit.)* It was all fine. *(Good.)*

I am still scared about having a baby though. I really don't know if I've made the right decision? I don't feel like the mothers in the movies at all. You know…like when the wife holds up the pregnancy test which reads positive and the couple embrace and everything is peachy! I feel petrified and completely unqualified. I have dreams, and I thought nothing could ever get in the way of those dreams. But a little sperm has. He swam straight past that rubber diaphragm and changed my destiny. There is just so much I want to accomplish, and now everything is ruined. I have to put my life on hold, even this new pop group I am signed with. *(Well, I'm not actually signed with them, it just sounds cool to say I am.)* We are called 'Glamrock', because we are absolutely glamorous and we rock *(ha ha)*. Our first single is coming out soon. However, how can I be a pregnant Diva? Shit, shit, shit. I am going to have to tell them really soon, although Adele told me to wait 12 weeks to do this. I am quite sad, come to think of it. I'm going to have to leave the group, even though

JC constantly tells me that the group is so trashy and way too 80's...

But then again, I think that's why I love it.

WEEK 7

14 October

Wow, I had absolutely amazing sex this morning. You've got to love the fact that you don't need to use contraception when you're pregnant. However, afterwards I just burst into tears. I think it's because I don't want things to change. Everything feels so fantastic between JC and I right now that I am having second thoughts. I really don't want to lose what we have.

Please God, let them stitch me up tight.

15 October

Today arrived the first copy of Glamrock's CD single 'Crucified'. The song originally released by 'The Army of Lovers' back in the 80's. And our single is already No. 6 in the Polish dance charts and No. 10 in Sweden.

I am on the front cover looking absolutely unbelievable. (*Like a hooker with a bad hairdo.*) Even so, I am overwhelmed with excitement. I cannot believe it; I feel like a real pop star.

We are Abba in dominatrix leather (*minus one girl*). I know it's tacky, but I love it. I almost peed my pants when the producer handed me the single. I have wanted my own

CD ever since I was 10 years old… I haven't told them I'm pregnant yet. Fuck it. For now I refuse to feel like anything other than a star.

16 October

Life sucks today. JC is a bit stressed out, and I really feel for him. I guess he has been dealing with a lot lately - work, being a supportive husband and of course the prospect of becoming a father. He was almost crying today, asking me whether our lives would still be the same. Would we still have careers? Were we making the right decision? To be honest, I have been thinking the same things. I am scared too.

I wonder if every couple feels this scared? Or just the ones whose contraception didn't work?

19 October

It's raining outside, as well as in my heart.

JC and I have been arguing. There is so much stress around us right now and we seem to be fighting every second of the day. I guess we are both scared and dealing with our insecurities in our own ways, but I hate fighting. It's awful. Deep down I keep thinking that if these fights go on, we will lose the baby. I am so emotional, and I just feel fucked. I am confused, happy, anxious and sad all at the same time. I am still not sure about having a baby and I just cannot seem to make peace with the decision. Why? Why? What's wrong with me?

I know I will be a fantastic mother and JC will make a great dad but our fights turn me off becoming a parent at all. We are in love and get along amazingly, but we fight miserably.

We misunderstand one another. It's almost as if we speak different languages *(which I know is partly due to the nine year age difference.)* This just leads to greater miscommunication and frustration. I yell, then he yells, then I scream, then he screams. Then he walks out and I feel like I want to punch his bloody face in. Yesterday I kicked and broke a really nice vase. I also threw a boot at his head. I can't believe it. This is not me at all. I am not a violent person, regardless of how good it feels to let it all out.

21 October

We have decided that we need to take a holiday. We are going to Australia for three weeks. I am so excited. I finally get to take JC home to meet my family and friends. It will be so wonderful.

I went in to see Mrs Z today about flying for 24 hours and she said there would be no problem at all, just to take my 'Mother Pass' with me to Oz, along with my folic acid and other supplements. She also suggested that I get a pair of thrombosis tights.

A pair of what?

22 October

I found a medical shop today who stock thrombosis tights. They are so ugly, and so tight. They aren't like proper tights either; they are two separate tights, like leg warmers pulled all the way up.

Not cool, but I am very excited about the trip.

23 October

I told 'Glamrock' today that I am pregnant. Surprisingly they were fine about it, they even said I could stay in the band and thought it might be cool for the group to have a pregnant singer. I told them it wouldn't be cool at all. I'm not going to look like Demi Moore when I'm pregnant as I have pigmy blood lines.

24 October

<u>A Poem</u>

When the baby comes, everything will change; I just won't feel like me,

I will be breastfeeding and changing nappies that are full of poo and wee.

When the baby comes, I probably won't have time to wash or dry my hair.

Will I even have time for a nice long bath? Does anybody care?

When the baby comes, the house will be dirty, and I won't have time to cook.

So what will I eat? When can I shop? They don't say THAT in the book.

When the baby comes will I be able to walk? I just might have to cry.

Cause my fanny might have split from the top of my clit right down to my left inner thigh.

When the baby comes my tits will be massive, and my boobies will probably sag,

I will breast feed till my nipples are raw, and I still can't have a fag!!

When the baby comes one thing is for sure, my life is going to change,

I know for a while the life I'm living will be so different and strange.

When the baby comes, I'm gonna be a mother, it's gonna be so great,

A tiny little beautiful person, and to be honest, I really can't wait.

25 October

JC and I took a long walk today, and as we were walking across the traffic lights I said; "Babe… Why don't we get married in Australia?"

JC stopped dead in his tracks and almost got hit by a school bus.

26 October

So… We have decided to get married. We always knew we wanted to. We thought about doing it this way because I do not get to go home very often and we want to have two weddings. One in Australia *(on the beach)* and one in London *(in the cold)*. We want to do it on the 8 November- that's almost three weeks away.

I wonder whether we can pull it off.

I wonder what my parents will say.

I wonder if I can wear stilettos in the sand.

28 October

I am writing this as I sit on the plane to Australia. We have been flying now for about four hours and I am not only bored but also completely uncomfortable. It's these fucking thrombosis tights. I feel like they are cutting off the circulation in my legs. Maybe I bought a size too small? I cannot believe that I have to wear them for another 19 hours. How can I get out of this?

Apparently I'm prone to thrombosis (being preggas.) If I take them off will I have to have my legs amputated *(or something?)*

And God I hate economy. I want to be famous right now. I want to be sitting in First Class feeling glamorous, instead of a fat ballerina squashed in the wings of a dirty old theatre.

29 October

We are in Singapore now. Two nights just to break up the flight. I love it here. It is gorgeous. Taking off my thrombosis tights as soon as we landed was even more gorgeous. What an unbelievable sensation! Such relief. The weather in Singapore is amazing: hot and humid, which I love. Our hotel is wonderful. Breakfast this morning was amazing. I am definitely hungrier being pregnant. Or is it just that I can let myself go? *(Something I haven't been able to do since I decided to be a performer.)* Our body clocks are completely out of whack however, and after we ate breakfast we went back to sleep for about seven hours, missing most of the day. We then woke up around 5pm and went out for dinner *(more food)*. Then went back to sleep at 11pm only to wake up at about 4am hungry again. Oh my god, I'm actually boring myself writing this…

29 October

We went to the markets today which were fabulous. We also spent about three hours swimming in the pool. We were doing back flips into the water and seeing who could do the perfect dive. *(I think I was the best.)* Need to sleep now as we leave for Sydney in the morning, Yipeeeeee!

30 October

Our flight is over. We are now in Sydney and it is so stunning. We have hired a four wheel drive and are staying in a small hotel near Neutral Bay. It's gorgeous, but we are both absolutely knackered and have been sleeping most of the day. I am so tired being pregnant. I'm sure I'm ten times more tired than JC. *(Even though he seems to whine ten times more.)* I really didn't realise I would get this tired. Pregnancy is hard work. I thought that all pregnant women did was eat ice cream and masturbate?

I have to get a wedding dress tomorrow.

31 October

I have found a hat. Well, it's a start. It's a fabulous vintage hat that I discovered in a second hand store. It's made of satin with a net across the face. Since it's a bit yellow I'm going to bleach it to try and make it white. *(Fingers crossed)*.

I talked to mum today and she asked me how my morning sickness was. I don't think I've ever had any morning sickness. I must be lucky.

1 November

We went to see some friends in the musical 'Footloose' tonight and afterwards I met a few of them at the stage door.

I was so nervous. I don't know why. Because I'm pregnant maybe? Deep down I felt like a fraud. I'm not qualified at all to become a mother. Come on, who am I kidding?

My friends love me for being funny and entertaining, lively and ambitious, driven and inspirational. Focussed on my career. Not a boring, old, domesticated mother!

I feel like an amateur. I mean, I don't know a thing about babies, or motherhood, being a parent, or raising a child? It's as foreign to me as, well... becoming a monk. My friends have never heard me talk about becoming a mother. I don't feel that it's cool. Maybe it will be, but at the moment it is <u>not</u> cool to have a baby. It has taken me over a month to convince myself that I should have one   at all, let alone be cool about it.

My friends were brilliant. They were so lovely, especially the girls. I didn't realise that so many women get so clucky over babies. I certainly never was.

It was such a relief, I must say. I really thought everyone might judge me, but they were all amazing.

The only person doing the judging was me.

2 November

I have found a dress. It was designed by fairies and it's gorgeous. It is very soft, made of silk and chiffon and such a loose fit my little tum doesn't stick out. *(I am getting a bit porky around my middle now.)* It's stunning and looks quite 40's. It will go with my hat perfectly. Yeah.

5 November

We arrived at my parent's house in South Australia late last night. I love their house. It's right near the beach - beautiful.

It is great to see my family, and they finally met JC *(whom my dad says reminds him of himself when he was young - 'tall, good looking and poor'.)*

My parents are really excited about the baby and are looking forward to having a fourth grandchild. It's really nice to be able to share some of the experience with them- even if it is only for four days. They are ecstatic about the wedding too. *(They won't have a bastard grandchild.)* Mum is being very motherly, organising wedding plans and making sure everything is perfect. Bless her.

To be honest, I don't even really feel pregnant anymore. I haven't been tired these last few days and I feel almost normal besides my little pot belly that is, which I'm hoping won't get any bigger before the wedding in three days.

7 November

We went out with my best friends from high school tonight, and after dinner they decided to give JC and I our wedding/baby gifts early. We were absolutely spoiled with baby blankets, clothes, books, toys, and some wonderful advice; "Have as much sex as you can now before the baby arrives."

I will have to keep that in mind. Thanks guys.

Oh shit, I'm getting married tomorrow.

8 November

WEDDING DAY

9 November

Well, yesterday was the most beautiful day. The weather was amazing, the day was perfect and everyone had a great time. Oh, and my heels looked great on the beach.

My dad walked me down the beach while JC waited with my family and a heap of strangers he didn't know. *(Bless him.)* We had loads of photos taken. I just hope my boobs don't look too big. I didn't realise how massive they are now. Afterwards we all went back to my parents' house, to a back yard reception. We had a BBQ, made a few speeches and sang a few songs. JC and I even put on our roller skates and did a couple of routines. *(I changed out of my dress for that.)* At about 11pm the limousine came to collect us.

Everyone was crying. And it was extremely hard to leave. Today we fly back to London, and it's so painful knowing that my family are not going to be around me while

I'm pregnant. It's not fair. Still, life goes on. Thank God for the internet and cheap overseas calls.

Anyway, we got back to our beautiful hotel with all our luggage and flowers from the wedding around midnight. I was on my back with my legs in the air all night. *(We couldn't find a vase!)* Bad joke. Goodnight.

11 November

We are in Singapore again - only for one night. I am feeling quite sick at the moment, as if I have period pain. Sometimes I feel a short stabbing feeling in my tummy. I guess the baby is getting bigger now as it's almost three months old. I hope this isn't how it's going to feel like for the next six months?

I am quite excited about having a baby now. I think I have had sometime to get used to it. And, well, I feel better. My family were able to meet JC. Now we are creating our own little family. What a wonderful new life we are going to have.

12 November.

The flight home was absolutely exhausting. 24 hours on a plane is just too long. However, my tummy felt much better the whole way home- which was great. My legs, on the other hand, were so swollen underneath my thrombosis tights that it was probably a good thing that I couldn't see my fat ankles. Otherwise I might have tried to jump out of the plane!

After touching down in Frankfurt, we boarded a train to our hometown. I was dreaming of sleep, a giant sleep in my own bed. Only three hours to go. Finally at two in the morning we stepped through our front door, Wow… the relief. I was so exhausted I fell straight to sleep.

At 7am in the morning, I woke with a really bad pain in my stomach. This was the same pain that had plagued me in Singapore but this time it was more intense and it just didn't feel right.

So of course the most rational thing to do was panic. I woke JC and told him about the pain. He was instantly frantic. I raced up out of bed to grab my encyclopaedia of baby books from the shelf to find out what might be happening. Then the pain got worse, and worse. It felt like very bad period pain. I was so scared, although I kept telling myself; "Kelly, you will be fine, everything is fine, don't be silly, you will see, you have nothing to worry about."

I miscarried four hours later.

Chapter 2

The Honeymoon is definitely over

"How can you grieve for something you have never seen?"

Kelly O'Brien

13 November

I am sitting in the hospital now waiting for my husband to pick me up and take me home. I feel like I'm in a dream. I can't believe what has happened? Everything was so perfect. How could this happen, God? Why? I feel empty. I feel silent inside like I don't know what to tell myself.

Kelly the eternal optimist. What a load of crap!

I want to cry. I want to lie in my bed and sob. This isn't fair. Why has this happened? Our baby was 12 weeks old, and now she is gone. Just like that. What did I do wrong? Was it the hot spa I had in Australia? Was it the dive I did off the pool in Singapore? Was it something I ate? Does God hate me? I thought my life was so perfect, but it's not. Everything is ruined. What do I do now?

The pain I felt yesterday was the most excruciating I've ever felt in my life. It was so horrible. I was screaming so loudly, as they pushed me down the corridor of the hospital. I can't believe I was in that much pain. The doctors said I was having contractions because my womb was trying to expel the foetus. Still… I thought pain like that could only exist in childbirth.

What do I do now? Who can I talk to? Who could possibly know how I feel?

I feel embarrassed for ever being pregnant. I mean- did I really think I could pull it off? I was kidding myself that I could be a mum. I feel so stupid, I feel so betrayed, so pissed off.

I want my baby back.

16 November

I cannot cry anymore. I am sick of crying. In fact, I think I've been crying too much. It's as though I am making myself cry because I feel I should. But now there are no tears left. My mind is trying to be so strong and block out the pain, I can feel it. My head has been really dizzy, I've been getting headaches and my eyesight is blurred. I can't concentrate on things very well, and sometimes I have pain in my stomach.

I can only be who I can be, and do what my body wants to do, but I don't know if I am doing this right.

17 November

I keep replaying the miscarriage in my head, I can't help it. I keep thinking that if I wish hard enough I can change what happened. But I know I can't.

I remember sitting on the toilet and looking down to see blood. At that moment I knew it, I knew something was wrong. I knew I had lost the baby. I remember crying uncontrollably and hoping, praying, that I was in a dream. Then we called a friend who took us to the hospital, the wrong hospital, where they weren't equipped to deal with miscarriages. The nurses put me on a drip *(which took six attempts)* and sent me off in an ambulance to a hospital for women. I can't remember the journey because I was in so much pain. Physical pain and emotional pain. I didn't have a baby anymore, but I was still in so much pain. For nothing. It was all for nothing. When I arrived, the staff wheeled me down the corridor and said they were going to do an ultrasound to check if there was a heart beat, but I knew there wouldn't be. My baby had no heartbeat and I felt as though my heart had stopped beating too. My baby was dead.

I was then taken into surgery where a nice doctor said; "It's alright Kelly, in ten seconds the pain will be gone." And he was right. I woke up later that day not feeling any pain- just completely empty. I had lost something I had never felt. Nobody can understand that, nobody but me.

19 November

Everyone knows what has happened. Friends have been calling to talk to JC asking how I am. It's nice to know that I have people in my life that care. However, miscarriage is just so hard to talk about. Nobody really knows what to say.

Mum, Dad, and my two sisters sent me a huge bunch of flowers today with a card that read; "We love you and we are thinking of you every day." I burst into tears when I read it. I wish they were here.

24

I went to see Mrs Z yesterday. She was really sad for me, but positive that in a few months I will be able to try again. She said that I would need about three weeks off work, but then I should go back as soon as I feel ready, to take my mind off things. I guess she's right. Starlight have told me to come back to work whenever I want.

One day at a time.

20 November

It's been a week now since the miscarriage, and I am doing OK.

I have been taking it easy, looking after myself, being gentle with my thoughts and trying to "tune into my sorrow." *(Well, this is what Louise Hay tells me to do.)* It's harder than it sounds.

I am trying so hard to relax and surrender, although deep down I know that I still have pain inside that wants to escape. JC has been wonderful. He too is emotional and dealing with the miscarriage in his own way. God, it must be so difficult for him, because he feels as though he needs to be strong for me while being so sad himself, and he's still working every night!

I have been feeling so many emotions. All the hormones that swam through my body when I was pregnant are slowly dissolving. That is why I feel so disjointed now. JC and I are adamant that we want another baby. However, the doctors at the hospital have told us to wait for three months before trying again as my body must heal *(along with my mind)*. We will wait.

I feel empty, but the same in a sense. I did not have much of a bump, nor did I see myself pregnant. Now I look no different than before. But before I f<u>elt</u> pregnant - it was like having eaten a warm piece of apple crumble. Now I don't feel the apple crumble. I just feel horrible.

22 November

Today I had a breakdown. I was doing OK. But then early this morning I accidentally wiped everything off my laptop.

I wiped it all. My emails, my friends addresses, personal letters, everything!!!

I was crying hysterically for hours. I just kept crying and crying. I completely lost it. I feel so sad, and now I feel like I'm not even sure if I want another baby. I don't know anything anymore. I'm so sick of everything. I really don't know what I think. I am feeling so sorry for myself that I feel as though I just want to fall asleep and die. I am so alone right now.

23 November

Feeling all right today. Although I can't help but wish that things were still the same as they were. It felt so beautiful being pregnant… but I'm not any more and that's the reality.

I spoke to Adele today. Her baby is due soon and I am so happy for her. But I feel a little sad as well that we couldn't be pregnant together *(even for a few months)*. She said she is huge and has 43-degree-days in Australia to put up with, poor thing. She said she feels like the Stay Puft marshmallow man from the first Ghostbusters film, slowly melting (but not actually white, or two hundred feet tall).

25 November

Last night JC and I had a terrible fight. I got awfully drunk on Sangria at a friend's going away party and started arguing with him. I was screaming, accusing and basically being a complete bitch. I feel terrible now; I was sooooooo over-emotional and a mess. I admit now that it was entirely my fault. I couldn't help myself at the time. I was upset and drunk, and you get like that when you're upset and drunk!

Then after you get upset and drunk, you run away down the high street, crying and sobbing and feeling sorry for yourself, thinking how wonderful it would be to be hit by a bus or a train and taken to hospital, where you would lie in critical condition, or even in a coma, for a few days so everyone else would feel sorry for you.

Why was I like this? Well… I guess I wanted sympathy really. I wanted JC to realise how fucking terrible and alone I felt. Which I'm sure he knew. But I wanted more attention, I wanted him to come running after me. I wanted him to tackle me to the floor while I was crying hysterically, then wrap me in a blanket and take me home where he would stroke my hair all night, telling me everything would be OK.

Instead, I ended up breaking my 8-inch stilettos, losing my purse and vomiting in my hair, before catching a taxi home where I was told off by JC for being stupid for running off. "Anything could have happened to you, why didn't you call me?" Oh yeah, I also lost my mobile phone.

26 November

Well today is a new day, and it started off beautifully. Firstly we woke up and had some fantastic sex. *(Why does this always happen when you have a hangover?)* JC wouldn't kiss me. *(I wonder why?)*

Then we walked through the Christmas markets, because of course it's November!

It was a beautiful day. We drank Glue wein, which is just like mulled wine *(except it tastes a bit like goat's breath with a hint of gasoline)*. Nevertheless it's quite potent and strong enough to kick-start the engine of a small aircraft. Very good. Then we went for a ride on the Ferris wheel, next to the ice rink. The Christmas markets are a completely bizarre concept for me. In Australia, at Christmas all we do is stay indoors (because it's too damn hot to go anywhere) drink cold beer and play Canasta….

Yes, Christmas in Germany is amazing; it really feels like Christmas here. *(So this is what all you Europeans talk about?)* OK, so now I admit it, Christmas in Australia is shit compared to here. *(There, I bloody said it. Happy, Claude?)*

27 November

JC and I went bowling with the cast last night. It was the first time I had really seen anybody since the miscarriage, so it was a bit weird. It was a 'themed' bowling night and everyone divided into teams and had to dress up. That part was exciting because JC's team dressed as 'Dead Rock Stars'. He chose Kurt Cobain, so I was able to see him in one of my dresses- very cool. I didn't dress up or play however, as I've been told to take it easy. *(Boring.)*

It was really strange seeing everybody for the first time. Nobody quite knew what to say to me. I guess it's hard to just come up and start a conversation. Most people were just really nice and supportive, asking if I was alright. This was lovely. There were others though who pretended like nothing had happened, which pissed me off at the time. One guy even asked me how the baby was. To which I replied; "Do I look <u>that</u> fat?" *(He felt awful once I'd told him the little tiger was in heaven.)*

I think it is hard for a lot of people to talk about something like miscarriage, because unless you've experienced it, or have had a partner or close friend who has experienced it, you don't know where to start.

Personally, I would have just preferred people ask me about it openly. I'm exceptionally honest and quite brash and I think it's better to talk about life's misfortunes than pretending something never happened, or chatting about the weather or what kind of bloody perfume you are wearing.

I honestly wanted my friends to ask me about the pain and ask me about the loss, ask me if it hurt, and if I cried non-stop for seven days. That would have been so much better. Miscarriage is something that so many women go through in their lives yet hardly anyone chats about it openly. Shouldn't we be able to talk about one of life's fucked-up tribulations? I think we should. And anyway, I hate bowling.

28 November

I had another big fight with JC. I don't even know what it was about but I feel terrible. Things seemed to be going so well after the miscarriage. We were both feeling OK and getting on with life. Now however, it seems we have lost our patience with each other. JC is annoying me and I'm sure he feels like I'm being a massive bitch!

The thing is, I'm sure we are like this because we both still feel vulnerable and hurt from losing our baby, but we can only feel how we feel at the moment. I guess we must try and be more patient and have a little more compassion for each other, but it's just so hard when he's being such a fuck-head.

29 November

I'm back from a girls' night. It was great. Just what I needed in fact, and it was a REAL girls' night; the kind of night where you talk about everything - cellulite, boob jobs, eating no carbs after 10am, lesbian affairs, getting tampons stuck up your minge, the works. It was great and so much fun.

My friend Kim was there tonight. She is six months pregnant and looks so beautiful. The moment I saw her I almost burst into tears; she seems so happy and tranquil.

It made me want to be pregnant again straight away, however JC is being such a prick right now, that sex with him is definitely not high on my list of priorities.

3 December

I miss being pregnant.

6 December

Adele is overdue; she still hasn't popped her baby out and is extremely over it. She said she can hardly manoeuvre herself around anymore and has to get Matt to tie her shoelaces because she can't reach at all. To add to her discomfort she is faced with 45 degree days, and is exhausted looking after her two other children, Jazzy (aged four going on twelve) and Levi, who is almost three. She must feel like poo.

7 December

JC has decided to take me to Paris so we can have some special time together. I am so excited. Oh my God I've never been to Paris. It will be so wonderful to get away for a few days, as I guess we never really had a honeymoon. We only had a miscarriage. *(OK, bad joke…)*

I have actually been feeling quite wonderful lately and this morning decided to shuffle and pick from a pack of fairy cards I have. *(They are always a welcome source of mystic information.)*

I picked 'Awakening your true self'. The explanation says; "You're beginning to recover your natural identity, including your old sense of humour, interests, passions and desires. Trust that any confusion or changes you're currently experiencing are part of your healthful evolution. As if a cloud has lifted from your mind and heart, you're beginning to see life and perspective of your old self. Now your old self is back!!"

Yeah, my old self is back, the fairies said so. Mind you, if I got a card I didn't like I would have done best out of three.

8 December

Well after quite an ordeal - we waited in the freezing cold at 5:30am for a train that never came - we are finally on the train bound for Paris, two hours late.

So right now I am sitting here in first class- one of the perks from having been screwed over this morning- with a glass of red wine. *(Yes, I know it's only 10 am but I'm on holiday.)* I'm listening to French people speak to each other across from me. *(I know, very bizarre considering we are in fact headed for Paris.)* Nevertheless I am incredibly excited. JC is asleep next to me drooling and I am enjoying the train ride.

Since the miscarriage I have been so up and down. I have felt completely depressed at times and completely elated at other times- a bit like taking ecstasy but having the come-down first. Very strange really. However, now I feel as though my spirit has lifted a little, like I've sprung back to life a bit more. JC and I haven't really spoken much about trying for another baby yet. We are mainly focussing on each other at the moment. In another few months we will talk about it. For now though, I need to wipe the drool off my husband's chin so people don't think he's dysfunctional.

9 December

Paris is beautiful. We are having such a gorgeous time. It's so great to relax, unwind and ease my mind *(sounds like a song)*. We saw the Eiffel tower yesterday, which is just so incredibly like the movies. But talk about freezing, fuck! My silicon boobs were turning into snow cones. I've never felt weather so cold in all my life. We also went to the Pere LaChaise today, a beautiful cemetery full of famous dead people. JC was very excited to be visiting Jim Morrison's grave, and for the occasion he whipped out a joint to pay homage to the dead rock star. I didn't indulge in a puff as I am not too good on the old weed. I am fine for about half an hour, laughing, giggling, chatting away, being a bit of a wanker. Then, however, the walls close in. I become paranoid, my mouth becomes drier than a nun's nasty, and I cannot stop eating for 36 hours straight. Yes, this is the fastest way for me to become an obese statistic. When I was 18 years old, I smoked non-stop for about two years and put on about two stone. I looked like a giant Cabbage Patch doll.

10 December

Last night, we went to the infamous Moulin Rouge, and it was quite spectacular - half naked girls, amazing costumes, lots of gay dancers pretending to be straight, and a three course meal...

I especially liked the woman who swam around in a see-through pool with two boa constrictors. How do women get into these professions?

Looking at all those naked women made me want to run to the bathroom and throw up the frog's legs I had just eaten; the women were all so thin. *(However their boobs were very small, so that made me feel better for about 37 seconds.)* Truth be told, these semi-naked, sequined girls reminded me how fat I really am.

Since the miscarriage I feel like I am still carrying amniotic fluid around with me everywhere I go. Why haven't I shrunk back to a size ten yet? Damn my body! Why doesn't it just do what I want? I want to feel slim and sexy again. I felt wonderful having a podgy belly when I was pregnant, but I'm not pregnant anymore, and I want those podgy bits gone…

11 December

Adele has popped out a little baby boy. Well plonked it out would be more correct *(cos he ain't that little)*. The beautiful, heavy little nugget weighed 9 pounds, 13 ounces and his head circumference was 38cm. Ouch, ouch, ouch. Adele also had a completely natural childbirth (for the third time). *I told her she should run for Prime Minister.* Adele and Matt have named their son 'Noah'. I asked her if the birth was OK, and she said; "We've filmed it, so you can watch it if you like."

"Ahhh, no thanks, not right now," I said. "I'm feeling way too glamorous having just got back from Paris…"

17 December

It is my first show back tonight, and I am so scared. I have butterflies in my stomach and I know it is going to hurt.

'Starlight Express' *(or 'Star Fright Depressed' as I want to call it now)* is a musical written by Andrew Lloyd Webber in the 80's. (You can tell by the costumes.) It is performed on a three story set, seats 1750 people and is the hardest job I have ever done in my life. We dance on roller skates, do back flips on roller skates, beat each other up on roller skates, and would probably fuck on roller skates if the show was still running in another 100 years. To be completely honest, it's bloody hard, quite insane and a tiny bit dangerous. *(JC has already broken his face doing the show.)* Added to all this, I'm not really very keen on any kind of aerobic activity whatsoever. Back in Australia, if I ever did an aerobics class, my friend PJ and I would do half the class, sneak out then go straight to the pub. Nice.

It is a fantastic show *(to watch)* and I am happy to be in it, regardless of the fact that I am going to wet my pants tonight *(after I vomit and shit myself)*.

18 December

My first show back was actually not as bad as I thought it would be. I built it up so much in my mind that I had scared myself half to death before I even got on stage. It was fine though. I was fierce, and it's good to be doing the show again. I love to sing and I forgot how much I had missed performing.

19 December

I went out to buy a pregnancy test today, as I've not had my period since I miscarried. So I got the test, did it, but the bloody thing didn't work, I got shafted.... I should have bought two! I'm pretty sure I'm not pregnant, however, I just wondered because I feel I should have had my period by now as I want to go back on the pill.

I think a part of me would love to be pregnant again, because of what I lost, but I know we can't. We're not allowed to get pregnant again so soon, and JC and I haven't even talked about it. I guess we have plenty of time to have a baby.

20 December

I am getting knackered already. Oh my god, the show is hard. *(Although my ass is getting harder, which I like.)* We have the Christmas Party to go to tomorrow night, so I guess that will be fun.

22 December

Great Christmas party. It was so wonderful to get dressed up and look gorgeous. It felt great to be out.

The party itself was completely amazing. When we walked in, the hall was set up like the North Pole, German-style. There was also candy floss, fresh ginger bread, crepes and sweets, German beer, and even fake snow falling from the ceiling. It looked incredible. I got drunk very quickly and was having such a fantastic time. I think I really needed to let it all out; it was exactly what the doctor ordered *(Not literally of course.)*

I also got quite pissed quite quickly (didn't eat enough ginger bread obviously.) I then proceeded to have a couple of lines of coke. Very spontaneous… I thought; "Fuck it, what the hell?" Anything to bring the old Kelly back to life…

Then "Oh my God", talk about chatty...

Ijustkepttalkingandtalkingandgoingonabouteverydam nthingIcouldthinkof, musthaveboredthepantsoffwhoeveritwa sIwastalkingtoo.WhowasItalkingto?

It was a wonderful night. I even got up and sang "Lady Marmalade" with the band and was a big hit.

JC and I had a nice long talk about everything. Having another baby, doing another year with the show, and how much we love each other *(lots)*. It was great *(It was also good coke!)*

We both decided that we are going to focus on each other for now, as we think that having another baby can wait a little while, maybe even a few years. We are so in love and want to spend all our time together right now. We also decided that we would both like to do another year at Starlight, and then maybe after that we would think about a baby.

Got home about 3am, couldn't sleep, had lots of sex.

23 December

JC's mum Sylvia arrived today from London. She is staying for a week over Christmas, and she's absolutely lovely. It's great having her here. Although we will be doing a show on Christmas Day, so that kinda sucks. The Germans celebrate Christmas Eve here, so we get tomorrow night off instead, and are going to see Sylvie's good friends Sue and Michael who live not far from us in Germany.

25 December

Christmas was great. We ate so much food, opened some great presents and danced all night long to 'Fleetwood Mac'. To be honest, I was quite exhausted. I've been feeling really tired lately. I think it's because I am back doing the show.

I missed my family so much today and was a bit sad actually. I missed having a Christmas BBQ and eating champagne and pancakes for breakfast. I missed opening presents in front of my parents and watching everyone get excited about their gifts.

I just missed being home.

Merry Christmas O'Bees.

27 December

I still haven't got my period, I am waiting patiently for it to come so that I can go back on the pill but it's not here yet. I guess my body has gone through quite an ordeal and my hormones have been pretty out of whack, but I hate using the withdrawal method with a young virile man; I don't think it's very safe. They say they can pull it out in time, but who really knows if they are capable of doing it perfectly? The pill will be a lot safer for me. And although I will put on a few hundred stone, at least I will have peace of mind.

31 December

New Year's Eve.

Well I can't say it was a quiet one. It was anything but. JC and I had a tremendous fight. For starters, I think New Year's Eve puts an awful lot of pressure on everyone in the world to have a good time; I mean, what if you don't feel like being happy and you end up having a miserable start to the New Year? Does that mean your whole year is going to turn out like shit? It's all too much *(and yes, I'm saying this because I had a crap time)*.

Firstly JC, Sylvia and I went out to a Thai restaurant with friends. It was quite cosy, great food, and wonderful conversation. I drank two massive Pina Coladas (which were gorgeous,) then five minutes to midnight we all went out onto the street with glasses of champagne and watched the fireworks.

Afterwards we planned on meeting friends at a nearby bar, but when we got there JC decided it was really not his kind of thing. It was like a gay sauna, with a perky pop DJ and a cocktail of freshly squeezed disco divas. *(I thought it was fabulous.)*

Everyone was completely off their chops on ecstasy, coke, LSD, German beer *(because that's almost as potent)* and, of course, the New Year's Buzz. However, before I could ask JC what he wanted from the bar, he had spat the dummy and walked out.

This lead to a screaming match on the street *(yes, very classy I know)*. I was extremely upset, more upset than usual, and when we got into a cab 15 minutes later I just cried and cried all the way home.

I got into bed at 1:10am. Crappy New Year!

1 January. 2005

JC and I made up this morning *(he apologised)* then asked why I was so emotional last night? He said he'd never seen me so upset about something so trivial. I said I didn't know why, and that I was probably just pre-menstrual…

Sylvia went home today, so JC and I spent the whole day snuggled up on a double mattress in front of the TV in the lounge making love, playing games and getting completely stoned. It was wonderful; and I let my appetite run riot. We ate pizza and apple strudel, chocolate, ice cream, sweets, toasted ham, cheese and tomato sandwiches and drank Baileys. It was gorgeous. Now I know I said I rarely smoke dope; however when I do, it's great. Food tastes great, sex is great, sleeping is great; being out of it just feels great... Nothing could have been better. We had such a wonderful time. The day was perfect.

2 January

Today I feel as though I am going to vomit every time I speak. I think I consumed my own body weight in chocolate last night.

3 January**

Something extraordinary has happened! I am pregnant *(again)*. It just seems completely incomprehensible. No wonder I have been feeling so strange. This explains everything. We just cannot believe it. I was only pregnant two months ago and we were told that after our miscarriage that we had to wait three months. *(I never was any good at obeying the rules!!)* JC must have some fast-swimming, potent young virile sperm in there, because we were being careful. Fuck me! Well, yes, apparently he did a good job of that.

We are so amazed, and very excited, but oh my god, the marijuana I smoked... The alcohol I've consumed, the cocaine I... Fuck, Fuck, Fuck. Oh shit. Do I tell the gyno? Will I be arrested? Am I a bad mother?

But I never knew. We were planning to wait. We also don't know if it's safe for me to be pregnant again so soon.

What if I can't have this baby?

What if I can?

Chapter 3

The Immaculate Conception

"It sometimes happens, even in the best of families, that a baby is born. This is not necessarily cause for alarm. The important thing is to keep your wits about you and borrow some money."

Elinor Goulding Smith

6 January

Firstly Mrs Z congratulated us on a job well done. I think she was actually just as surprised as we were! She then proceeded to take a look at what was going on down there. First she gave me an internal, then took a swab and proceeded to stick a nasty vibrator looking gadget up my foo. Then we all had a look on the screen at a tiny little blob which we were told was a six week old foetus. It looked fascinating, and to think only two weeks after my miscarriage I got pregnant again so soon. Afterwards, I gave some blood and we walked away feeling quite elated. We are so happy (and a little freaked out as well). We thought we wouldn't be having another baby for ages. We just can't believe it! We were not ready for this at all. However, I feel as though we have been truly blessed. What a miracle. Wow…

I am back at work now *(after having three weeks off after the miscarriage)* so I am going to have to tell them I am once again pregnant. They are going to think I got knocked up on purpose for sure… But I didn't I swear. *(Here I go feeling like a 12 year old again.)* I shouldn't feel guilty. What has happened is an amazing thing. I still can't quite comprehend it. How did this happen again so quickly?

JC's sperm should enter the Olympics. It would only take them three hours to swim from London to Greece.

WEEK 7

7 January

I am already in my seventh week of pregnancy. I can't believe it. I was 12 weeks pregnant not so long ago.

Maybe I never lost the baby at all? Maybe it was a mistake? But how can it be? This baby is just a pumpkin seed. The other one was the size of my big toe. I feel like the Virgin Mary. I have conceived immaculately.

8 January

It is weird being pregnant. I had got used to the idea that I wouldn't be a mama for a couple more years, and now this whole process is starting again. If I knew I was going to be pregnant again just two weeks after I miscarried I would not have got so drunk, smoked so much weed, cried so much or thought about being hit by a train!!!

Shit. I'm pregnant. Oh my God. I have to remind myself so I don't light up a big fat doobie to smoke just to cope with the weirdness of it all. And I look so normal... I wish I had a big fat stomach straight away. I want to at least LOOK pregnant, but it takes ages to get to that stage *(sigh)*.

I guess I will have to be patient, at which I'm not very good at.

Apparently the baby is now forming all of its vital organs. This is the time that is crucial to a baby's development- well that's what Miriam Stoppard *(the pregnancy goddess author)* says. So I am trying to eat very well and I have cut out all heavy spirits - I mean alcohol - from my diet. JC smokes, but he is not smoking anywhere near me. I really want to be aware of everything I need to know this time and do my best.

We have told our immediate family about our news *(again)* and they are so happy for us. We are not telling too many other people though this time until three months has passed and I am going to try and keep working at Starlight for as long as I can. Mrs Z said doing the show is fine. She said that even if I fell, the baby is so small and so supported in my tum *(probably due to all the fatty tissue)* that it would be fine. The show however is really hard. I am so tired on stage and I've been feeling rather sick as well. Hope I don't vomit all over my skates.

9 January

I am scared about having the baby again, not about losing it again (*although that has crossed my mind*) but losing myself. Being pregnant again is scary. It's like, right there... twenty centimetres below my breast bone, forming into a perfect baby as I write this. Yes (sigh) it's come back to this again. I'm completely thinking of myself. I'm totally selfish. What can I say...?

10 January

The show is so hard. I am feeling sick and very tired, and apparently women are prone to narcolepsy when they're pregnant. GREAT! Actually, now there's a funny story. When I first started rehearsals for this show, a girl named Chantelle told me she had narcolepsy. Being quite naive, and having no idea at the time what narcolepsy was I said; "Oh, my god, is that sex with dead people?" Anyway, she was not amused and proceeded to correct my medical terminology, advising me that narcolepsy means you can literally just 'nod off' any where, any time of the day. I will never forget the meaning of that word.

11 January

Well I have woken up this morning with quite bad morning sickness; I had it last night as well, which was very frustrating because as horny as I was I just could not have sex with my husband. I am going to call Adele for some quick fix remedies....

12 January

I am still working. I guess it's only been nine days, but I think I'm going to die! I have to tell them soon, the show is not getting any easier for me. I do a back flip in it for God's sake.

Oh, Adele said 'fresh ginger'.

WEEK 8

15 January

I just realised that I also need to tell the record company that I am pregnant again. Shit, Fuck, Poo. I think I'm too scared. Actually, I know I'm too scared. I'm rubbish!

But I have to tell them because I have to QUIT. I can't be a pregnant trashy slut bag. There are more important things in life that blonde wigs, fake lashes, and leather pants. And I only sing one verse in the fucking song anyway.

16 January

Oh my god, I am having anxiety attacks again. I keep thinking that we are not ready to have a baby. It feels right, then it feels wrong. I want a baby, then I don't. I want to be pregnant, then I'm petrified. I want to give birth, then I think; "AM I INSANE?"

I want to be a mother, yet at the same time I like my life how it is. I love being me and carefree, but I also want to experience a different side to life.

I still have so much I want to do. I want to work with great musicians, be a comedienne, perform in West End shows and be a Diva. I guess I still want to be <u>a star!</u> Let me make this perfectly clear: when I write about being a 'star', it's not necessarily the kind of star everyone automatically thinks of - no Britney Spears, Jordan or Christina A Gorilla. It's my own version, a unique vision I have of myself that makes me feel like I'm <u>a star</u>.

In my head I keep dreaming that I can do both. Be a wonderful mother and a star. But can I really? Is that possible? I guess I could be? I mean who is 'in charge' of my dreams anyway? There is no doubt in my mind that I can do both, but it will be hard, and I'm sure I will have to sacrifice a lot to pursue my dream of 'Supermum, Superstar', but deep down I think I can do it... Actually I know I can. And I will.

18 January

Tonight I put pillows up my t-shirt to see what I would look like pregnant, and I just looked fat.

21 January

We have told work that I am pregnant again. I felt so uncomfortable about doing this, and deep down I just wanted my mum to write a letter to my bosses telling them I was having a baby again. However I had to be grown up and just be honest... So boring! Once again though, they were completely understanding and supportive.

So I have stopped working again and now spend my free time reading about babies and how to become the perfect mother... ha!

I am really sad today. I miss my family in Australia. This is going to be such an amazing time for me and I wish I could share this with all of them. But I can't. I guess that I must experience this new adventure on my own.

I have started taking photos of myself *(or rather my expanding waistline)* to send back to family and friends in Australia. I am definitely going to keep in touch with emails and photos, as I'm sure everyone will be quite interested to see how kind pregnancy is to my body.

WEEK 9

22 January

We made our second visit to Mrs Z today and received all the results for all my tests. I am fabulously healthy. Oh, and we saw the blob again- although this time it had a tiny little heart beat, and two heads. *(Apparently the second head is known as the egg sack.)* We were told that the baby is looking good, and instructed to come back again in another month. Man, this is going to take forever…

Everyone keeps asking me if I feel pregnant. I say 'yes, absolutely, I've never felt so crap in my life'. Morning sickness sux. I feel like shit. I feel like I'm being punished for partying so hard in my early 20's.

23 January

<u>A poem</u>

Oh what a beautiful morning, the birds are singing outside,

I feel so happy being pregnant, it's a feeling that I just cannot hide.

It really does make me excited, I wish I were a clown that could laugh,

but I'm not, I feel awful this pain is exhausting, and to be honest I just want to barf.

I feel so sick in my tummy, and I think; "What the hell is this for?"

I can barely make it to the bathroom sometimes, never mind the bloody front door.

Morning sickness, yes it sounds cute at first, to be pregnant and big in the belly,

but it's not like that, I really don't feel like me, and my boobs droop down to my belly.

And the whole time you think that you can eat what you want,

so I eat loads of chocolate and candy.

But it makes me feel sick; this stuff tastes like shit,

What I want is a scotch or a brandy.

I want my husband to feel how I feel - awful and sick in the guts.

Maybe he would <u>really</u> understand, if I kicked him hard in the nuts?

Oh morning sickness bloody sod off, you make me feel so blue.

Isn't it enough that in seven months, my punaani will be tearing in two?

24 January

So many thoughts are filling my mind today. Pregnancy is fucking me up. I am analysing everything lately, because I know that very soon my life is going to change dramatically. It will probably seem as if I am a completely different person.

My relationship with JC is going to change too, and yes, I am petrified at times, because my life has always been fantastic. I have always been a happy person, an ambitious woman, a determined and talented performer, and my lifestyle has always been spent selfishly, looking only after myself.

However, we have decided to have a baby, and that means that for a change we will be looking after someone else. It's going to be so weird. Everything I've ever known is going to change, especially me. It will probably be like going through puberty again.

I do really want to be a mother. And I welcome the challenges that lay in store for me *(I am an Aries after all)*. I want to experience life through a different camera lens. I want to love a child and teach him or her what I know. I want to experience being a family, and the magic a child will bring into our life. I want to simplify my life by not worrying about things that don't really matter. I want to laugh more.

Deep down I know everything will be wonderful. I just think so damn much lately.

Being pregnant so far has been a head-fuck. I know as soon as I accept this decision to become a parent and feel at peace with it, I will enjoy it more. I guess that is just going to take time. It's like saying goodbye to your old self, and anticipating the arrival of the new. I guess I should feel blessed to experience such an amazing transformation.

25 January

I once heard that thoughts are like boomerangs. At the moment however, my thoughts feel like a frickin' Yo-Yo. I am OVER IT… I go from being totally excited about having a baby, to totally afraid. I am trying to convince myself that I am making the right decision, but to be honest, I'm still scared. I have no idea whether I'm making the right choice. God, I feel so pathetic. Usually I just go for it, jump right in and take chances with my life. However, this time it's different. This chance is going to change everything.

Please universe, give me some guidance.

26 January

Australia Day. (*Does anybody give a shit?*) I got up at 10:30 am, made some peanut butter on toast and had a gourmet coffee, which I've heard is kinda bad; however I love my coffee, it makes me happy, keeps a smile on my face, and I'm addicted to it. So shoot me!

I heard the song 'All that she wants is another baby' this morning and am wondering if that is the 'guidance' the universe is giving me?

In retrospect I guess the universe couldn't find a song called: 'I'm a selfish bitch, all I care about is me…'

27 January

I went for a swim tonight at the pool and saw two pregnant women there. I wanted to say something to them; "Wow, you're pregnant! Hey, so am I." But basically the only thing I can say in German is; "Can I have a latte? Can I order a taxi?" So I just gave them a friendly smile instead.

I think I will have to brush up on my German soon. I wonder how you say; "Give me a bloody epidural right NOW?"

WEEK 10

28 January

I feel absolutely awful. Today is a 2/10. I feel like shit. I am over tired. I have a terrible headache, my brain feels as though it is being squeezed between a vice and my eyes can't concentrate. To top this off, my husband is being a dick. He is completely misunderstanding me. I feel extremely vulnerable and lonely. Yesterday I was feeling so energetic and full of vitality. What happened overnight? It's like I've transformed from a butterfly back into a caterpillar.

Anyhow, tomorrow is a new day and my husband said he is going to give me a foot massage later while we watch a movie.

Gold.

30 January

I haven't told all my friends back home that I'm pregnant yet. I am going to wait until my first trimester is over this time. However, I am a little apprehensive about telling everyone again, as I feel like people are going to judge me and think I'm making a stupid decision. My friends back home have such huge expectations of me. They have all been so supportive regarding my singing career over the past ten years, and I really think they all believed *(as I did)* that I would become a big star over here.

Part of me feels like I am giving up. But I'm not. I have promised myself that I will never give up, I will always keep going. Entertaining is my life. I am just putting my career on hold for a while that's all.

I hope my friends will understand and keep believing in me… They have to.

2 February

Starting to feel a bit more confident about being a Supermum.

I guess that whatever I believe will be my reality, and that's what I must keep reminding myself. I can do whatever I want. I can have a baby and still be successful. Lots of women have done it.

WEEK 11

5 February

I just realised today that I probably won't be able to do any pre-natal classes here in Germany. My German is shocking, and I think you really need to be able to understand what is being said when people are referring to your vagutz.

My girlfriend Danni said I should be fine without them though, as I'm a singer…???

7 February

I am so sick this morning. I also felt sick last night, and actually come to think about it, I've been feeling sick for the last four weeks. Why does it feel so awful? I can't do anything. This morning sickness is awful business. I'm not throwing up, but I feel like I'm constantly hung over. I thought morning sickness would make me feel sick in my stomach, but it's more than that… I have lower energy, headaches, and just feel shit a lot of the time. And what's with the name morning sickness? I feel sick in the damn afternoon, at night time and even while I'm sleeping. Fucking morning sickness my ass.

9 February

I talked to my Mum and Dad tonight. They were having a midnight BBQ with friends in the beautiful warm Australian weather. I was so jealous. They are in the process of planning a trip to Germany after the baby is born. However my Dad says he doesn't want to fly and would rather go by ship. He hates flying. He said he doesn't even mind if it takes six weeks to get to Europe- he would still rather go by sea. So I told Dad that if he wants to be here just after the baby's born in September he will have to leave in July.

WEEK 12

12 February

I am now in my twelfth week but I still feel sick, although Mrs Z assures me this is a good sign, because women who experience nausea rarely miscarry.

I love nausea, I love nausea!

However, I have a band gig tonight at the Hilton Hotel, so I hope feeling poorly does not interfere with my rendition of 'Disco Inferno'.

13 February

I have just come home from my gig. It's 1:30am and I am freaking out. I have cramps in my stomach and I am so scared. It feels similar to the pain I had last time when I miscarried, except not as intense. The doctor is not open and I don't really want to go to the hospital. Maybe my tummy hurts from singing? But that's never happened before. All I can do to make myself feel better is write. I'm sure I am OK. I have to be. I am going to try and sleep now and I will go to the doctor tomorrow if it still hurts.

9am: Everything's OK. The pain has gone, and after talking to Adele this morning I realise that my tummy was hurting because I had been singing last night for four hours straight. Adele said that the muscles, joints and ligaments in your body when you are pregnant soften up and grow tenderer. Therefore if I am pushing from my diaphragm to sing, my stomach is obviously going to get sore. Phew! I'm so happy. I was very panicky last night. The gig actually went really great. I had so much fun *(even though I had a pot belly and people probably thought I'd just eaten too many pork pies).* When I got home however, I was in so much pain and just an absolute wreck.

I think it's because my only memory of being pregnant last time was having a miscarriage at 12 weeks and I am in the twelfth week now.

I was so frightened that it was all happening again and I kept thinking to myself; "I just can't go through this again God. Please!"

JC kept telling me to calm down and relax, but I'm pregnant, so rationality disappears. I feel so ridiculous now. However at the time I was almost convinced that something was wrong.

I even kept going to the toilet sure that I was going to see blood any moment. I was terrorizing myself. What a wanker!

I wanted to go straight to Mrs Z, but it was 2am when I got home. So I had to wait eight hours to see her, which seemed like an eternity to me.

I was doing everything I could do to take my mind off that terrible feeling. I took a bath, read a book, talked to JC. But nothing worked. I was scared out of my wits.

Then I calmed down a bit, lay down on my bed and began breathing slowly in and out, trying to imagine the baby being surrounded by white light. After a few minutes, I then realised that the baby was fine, instinctively I knew she was OK.

I finally got to sleep at around 4am, and woke up around 7am to call Adele, who should really have her own website www.calmestmotherintheworld.com   She is like a pregnancy guru and assured me that everything was fine. And she was right. I mean it all seems so logical now, but pregnancy and logic? Well they go together like salmon and ice cream. *(Oops, I think that just made me want to throw up.)*

14 February

Valentines Day!! I was very spoiled today. JC bought me some gorgeous earrings and a pair of the funkiest shoes I've ever seen. He is an angel. I wonder sometimes what I would do without him. Just having him here for me is a Godsend. When I'm ill he makes me ginger tea with honey and lemon, he massages my feet, runs me hot baths and fixes me gorgeous food to eat when I am knackered and can't to do anything for myself. I am so fortunate to have him, as I now realize how difficult it would be being on my own. Being pregnant can be so draining. Wow, I never thought it could take control of you like this. I am constantly a victim to my needs; if I need to sleep, I sleep, if I'm hungry I have to eat, and if I'm grumpy, well- HIDE! I get vicious. Beforehand I would have gone without sleep and food and I would have pretended I was cheery. You can't do that when you're pregnant. You have to honour every feeling. It's a kind of surrender, and quite nice in a way. I feel like a child; if I want something, I want it now. I don't think about my weight or how many calories I've eaten today, and I don't think I've ever done that in my life. It's bloody marvellous. And I try to honour my body as much as I can. For instance, if I want some cheese cake there must be a reason for it; I obviously need some calcium.

Chapter 4

Tits.......

"I used to rush to the mirror every morning to see if I had bloomed, but all I did was swell. My ankles looked like flesh-coloured flares and my breasts were so huge they needed their own postcode."

Kathy Lette

WEEK 13

19 February

I have had a headache for two days now, although it feels more like a migraine, and it has not subsided for a second. I thought all the pain would have stopped by now. I'm entering into the second trimester soon and I have been so excited, like getting through the first stage on a Game Boy. However, maybe God hates me and is going to make me suffer for this whole pregnancy?

And I still don't even know whether I am 12 or 13 weeks, and it's really annoying me. I always thought I was

13 weeks; however Mrs Z said that the baby looked a little smaller this month and then the computer worked out my delivery date was a week later than she first thought. That's soooooo not fair. Every week counts in this game.

I had eight girls from the show over tonight. I made Spaghetti Bolognese, Greek salad, and garlic bread, it was a big hit. Then we watched my old singing and dancing videos from when I was 11-years-old. They were very funny and the girls thought I was hysterical, which made me feel very popular. My friend Sarah also gave me a beautiful baby photo album with a gorgeous card that said; "Dear Kelly, I really can't believe there is a tiny baby inside you, that's just so amazing!" So sweet...

20 February

I have been staring at my boobs for about half an hour and I am afraid. Very afraid. They are already a D-cup, but seem to still be growing rapidly. What if they get so big that they just explode? Could they actually pop? I don't know. I really don't need them to get any bigger though, as I will just look like a knocked-up prostitute.

21 February

Bloody pregnancy. I thought that there would only be morning sickness. Wrong!

I have constipation and this awful feeling in my legs. It's like there is no circulation and they feel heavy, itchy and nasty. I'm calling them 'Itchy legs'. I hope it doesn't mean I'm going to get varicose veins like my girlfriend Kylie did when she had her first baby.

So I am lying in bed all day today. I think I need to relax and put my stomach up!

22 February

Food just isn't fun anymore. I used to love eating. Now it is such a chore and when I do eat it's a mission to keep it down. Fuck those women on the television who are gorgeous and pregnant, looking glamorous, asking their husbands to run down to the nearest 7-11 for some vanilla ice cream and a hot dog, what a crock of shit! And why are women still going to work? Why? Personally, I think all women should be sent off to a health retreat for nine months and be pampered like Cleopatra herself. *(Maybe not bathed in milk though as that would only make us barf.)*

24 February

I have humongous love handles. Why, God? Tell me? What do I need those for?

I mean, I can understand the big boobs, but enormous love handles? Come on…. When does this whole pregnancy thing become fun?

WEEK 14

25 February

I think I'm having a girl. I just have that feeling. I think because I gave my mum such a hard time when I was a teenager that Mother Nature is paying me back already. Yep, definitely a girl.

27 February

We have booked some flights to go to London on Monday. I am really looking forward to it. It's hard to write at the moment because I don't feel so good. I have these awful tingly heavy itchy legs again which I hate and I've barely been sleeping. I also keep farting. I know I need to be more positive, but I can't be. I'm tired and cranky and I need to sleep.

1 March

I am not happy *(again)*. I have been eating soldiers *(boiled runny eggs on slices of toast)* for the past 28 years. It is my favourite dish in the whole world. Now I have found out that eggs must be cooked all the way through when you're pregnant, as one in 450 eggs contains salmonella. Good one!

For starters I don't like hard eggs and more to the point - what if I've already contracted salmonella? I have probably eaten over 70 or 80 eggs in the time I've been pregnant and the baby is still safe and obviously happy. But how can I go on eating runny eggs now? If anything ever happened I would never be able to look another hen in the eye again. Now there's a great song....

(To be sung to the tune of 'You can't hurry love')

"I can't look at you. No, you just laid an egg...
It's got salmonella, I can't eat it, I'm so afraid....."
How long must I wait, (pause) to eat one again?
I'm having a baby, you are just a stupid hen!"

2 March

Today I am feeling more positive. Considering all I seem to be doing lately is complaining.

There is a lot that is pissing me off about being pregnant but I am getting used to it and I am starting to enjoy it. I certainly enjoy that I can eat whatever I want. And I am not working anymore. I'm happy being a little housewife and that I get to do all the things I've always wanted the time to do. I am also quite excited by the drama pregnancy creates. It's new. It's completely new and it's always amazing reading about my baby's progress. It's a special time, so I should be enjoying it more...

That's it. From now on I am only going to be positive!

3 March

Damn pregnancy!

I mean I know its God's creation of life and everything but the only creation I am seeing at the moment is my fat cells expanding, creating cellulite.

FAT! Where does it all come from when I hardly eat anything? Does the Fat Fairy fly in through my bedroom window at night and inject chocolate cake, cocoa pops, and last year's left-over Easter eggs into my ass for fun? I can feel myself getting fatter and fatter and I just don't like it. And yes, I know I am pregnant for God's sake, but I am still tortured. I actually found my old measurements today, and I almost cried. *(Actually I really did cry.)*

My measurements used to be:

Waist - 27 inches

Hips - 32 inches

Bust - 34.5 inches

Thighs (just one) - 20.5 inches

Now I measure:

Waist - 30 inches

Hips - 34 inches

Bust - 36 inches

Thigh - 21 inches

Okay, so the thighs are not so bad, but I feel like the rest of me is out of control. Why are there some women that only get a big bump on the front and nothing else? My girlfriend Danni was like this. She is tiny and when she was pregnant with her son Jacob she had a tiny cosmopolitan "Sex and the City" bump, the bitch! I can tell you right now - my body is not going to look cool. I'm going to look like a watermelon.

I can't actually believe that my body looks different already. I'm only in my thirteenth week and I am seriously losing my lovely voluptuous figure.

JC says I look exactly the same. But I DO NOT look the same. A girl knows her own body, and mine is different. I mean for starters, when I lie down on my back and pull my stomach in *(trying to look emaciated)* I can't see my hip bones anymore. Also, my tops are all too short now due to the swelling of my breasts (which are just going to look ridiculous soon.) I feel like a beached whale *(without the beach, and some fins, and rubber skin, and a blow hole)*. NO, I'm not taking this all too far. Oh *(I'm crying again)*. Why does it matter so much? I know I'm pregnant, but I just don't like it. I think I will feel much better when I have a big bump on my stomach, and then at least I will <u>look</u> pregnant. At the moment I just look like a sumo wrestler.

Nobody likes to feel out of control and unattractive. In the past, if my self esteem was ever down I would just go shopping, but that alone raises even more issues....

<u>FASHION!</u>

For starters, I just cannot open up another pregnancy book to see photos of expectant mothers wearing beige.

Beige - why this colour? Is beige the pregnant women of the world's international colour? Does it have something to do with us looking like marsupials? Or is it so that we might blend into our chocolate milkshakes? I mean, don't get me wrong, these women look nice, but not only are they all dressed in beige, they are all over 40 (not that there's anything wrong with that). But I'm in my twenties, and I refuse to wear beige… Or fucking leggings *(it's just so 1985)*. My jeans are getting so tight, and my denim doesn't really stretch. But what do I wear? I still want to look cool. I'm a cool chick. I have always looked good, and it's disgusting to face the fact that I may be looking like a Peacock's catalogue soon.

I must find new maternity fashion to wear, but where will I find FUNKY maternity fashion? And will it look good on me? Previously I only had to think about making my ass look smaller, now I'm going to have to think about trying to make EVERYTHING look smaller.

I mean, you spend a few years at the beginning of your twenties working out your own personal style, what looks good, what suits your body type, how wearing high heels is non-negotiable, only to find out when you're pregnant that all of this must change. *(N.B. I have not actually given up the heels yet. If I wore them on my wedding day on the beach, I can wear them while I'm pregnant.)*

Maternity wear….Hmmm, I've seen nothing yet that convinces me I should feel sexy being pregnant, not unless wearing a sleeping bag as a jumper is considered sexy. I'm not meaning to criticise the designers (I'm sure they do their best) but HELLO, not every pregnant woman is 39 years old, 6 ft tall, and has a long neck. I'm 5ft, a size 10 and my neck is short. I'm sure I am not alone here. Anyway, I have decided to steer clear of the maternity stores, and create my own pregnancy wardrobe…

<u>WEEK 15</u>

5 March

We have arrived in London today. I love it here. There is such a buzz and the people are amazing, so open minded, so diverse - and of course the shopping is incredible. I have also been told about a shop called 'Mothercare'. So I am hoping to find it.

I have actually started feeling a bit better today. I haven't had any morning sickness at all so far and have been feeling great. I am farting a lot though. Quite embarrassing really, especially when I was brought up to not fart at all. My Dad had three daughters, and was adamant none of us would ever fart- EVER! So, we got very good at holding it in. I know... It's unnatural, probably even illegal. And it's completely different now anyway, because I have no control over farting and it's humiliating. I don't like it. It's not ladylike. Yes, I have fart issues!

6 March

I have been thinking a lot about my career while I've been in London.

I think it's because I am surrounded by so many successful people here and it actually makes me want to vomit.

I also met one of JC's best friends for the first time yesterday. Her name is Victoria (Vix Bix) and she is stunning. *(She is also playing the fucking lead role in 'Oh What a Night!' at the moment.)*

Yes, well, I felt like a fat unemployed midget when I first met her. She is absolutely gorgeous, and really lovely. I shouldn't have felt weird and insecure around her really, but part of me just did. I felt so completely normal standing next to her; even though she did tell JC later that she thought I looked beautiful *(which was nice - thanks Vix)*.

8 March

I saw one of my best girlfriends in the world today- Roberta. She is the best and I love her. We met up in a bar and had a scotch and such a great chat. We have known each other a long time, as we lived close to each other in Sydney and became great friends. (*We also partied extremely hard together, which forms an inseparable bond!*)

I was a bit sad later on the tube ride home. I hope I still see my beautiful friends once I've had this baby.

10 March

I have been thinking about how wonderful it will be to finally live here in London. It's going to be amazing. This town is full of opportunities, and it's fabulous. *(As well as fabulously expensive!)*

But I don't feel as positive about my career as much as I used too. I feel like I've been setting my sights lower than usual. Which is sad because I used to have such amazing expectations of myself, such fabulous dreams; and now part of me feels as though I have to give up my dreams because I am becoming a mum.

Deep down I know everything else will have to take second place to our baby, including my career.

To me, having a baby means I have to give up being me. I hate that!!!!

Having a baby feels so realistic. Achieving my dreams now feels so unrealistic. I feel as though the magic in my life will be over once a baby is here. However, there must be women out there who have had children yet gone on to fulfil their dreams.

I am going to do some research and find some famous mother mentors. I am not going to let my dreams go. I have to make it happen. I must believe in myself and keep following my dreams, even if they have to be put on hold for a while...

I am going to do it too. Just watch me.

Didn't find fucking Mothercare by the way!

WEEK 16

12 March

We got back from London yesterday and it seems that my morning sickness has gone. I've not had it for a week now and I am soooo happy. I feel fantastic. I had so much energy in London; I rarely felt crap at all.

We went to see Mrs Z today. As usual I peed in a cup, got weighed and had my finger pricked. Ouch! Then we got to see the little bub, well, actually we didn't see much at all. Mrs Z just couldn't get a good ultrasound picture, and we only saw a fat blob. We were pretty disappointed. She said that next time it would be better as the baby would be bigger and we could probably even find out the sex too. Shit, I don't know whether I want to know the sex of the baby? I would like to wait until the big day but I'm so curious. Shit, Shit, Shit.

14 March

A Poem

When the baby comes, everything will change; I just won't feel like me,

I will be breastfeeding and changing nappies that are full of poo and wee.

When the baby comes, I probably won't have time to wash or dry my hair?

Will I even have time for a nice long bath? Does anybody care?

When the baby comes, the house will be dirty, and I won't have time to cook.

So what will I eat? When can I shop? They don't say THAT in the book.

When the baby comes will I be able to walk? I think I'm going to cry.

Cause my fanny might have split from the top of my clit right down to my left inner thigh.

When the baby comes my tits will be massive, and my boobies will probably sag.

I'll breastfeed till my nipples are raw, and I still can't have a fag!

When the baby comes one thing is for sure, my life is going to change,

I know for a while the life I'm living will be so different and strange.

When the baby comes, I'm gonna be a mother, its gonna be so great,

A tiny little beautiful person, and to be honest, I really can't wait.

16 March

Guess what? I found out that Reese Witherspoon had her first child when she was 22 years old, and... well she's still alive, happily working, married to that sexy Ryan Phillipe from Studio 54, and pregnant again, I think. They made it work. I mean, they have millions of dollars and can afford a good nanny, housekeeper, gardener, chauffer and a chef, but still - they make it work. *(Not now, they don't.)*

Then there's Judy Garland. She had Liza Minnelli when she was 24 years old, although I can't say she was much of a role model. OK, so let's scrap that one....

Who else? Still searching.

17 March

Today we found out the sex of the baby. I can't believe we did. We just couldn't resist. I was only originally going in to have another ultrasound to see how the bub was, but Mrs Z asked us whether we wanted to know the sex of the baby and I guess we are just two impatient kids...

I actually really wanted to wait to find out the sex, because almost every mother I've spoken to said that it is such a wonderful surprise to find out at the birth. But with the screen right there, right in front of our faces, and JC panting with excitement, I said "OK, tell us"

"Right... Well, there's one leg," Mrs Z said, "and there's the other leg, and that thing in between..."

"Is a damn big clitoris," I screeched.

"Is a penis," the doctor replied

"A boy?" I paused. "How can it be a boy? It's sooooo a girl." JC and I were both shocked. I had been thinking all along that I was having a girl; thinking of pink candy floss, princesses, Barbie dolls, sugar and spice and all things nice, not frogs and snails and puppy dog tails!

However, he's a boy, a gorgeous little smelly boy.

We are very happy though, of course we are. *(I would have been happy with anything vaguely human after the cocaine I took.)*

A boy! We didn't expect to be having a boy. However, we are really happy and now, somehow he feels like a real baby, not a cabbage patch doll. *(Yeah Kelly, like a cabbage patch doll would be trapped inside your womb for 14 weeks.)*

I feel so great today. I feel as though I am really going to become a mummy. For the first time it feels real, and OK, and really quite scary! Childbirth seems only weeks away.

I guess this is the part I have been waiting for; this is the happy part of the pregnancy, when the morning sickness is gone, I'm getting a big tummy, and I no longer feel the urge to treat my husband as a slave. Yes, pregnancy is bliss.

WEEK 17

18 March

I went out today and bought our first baby clothes- a pair of superman socks. They are for one month-old babies. Ha… better not blink!

19 March

J.K Rowling had her first daughter when she was 28-years-old. She was working on her Harry Potter books at the time. She hadn't even finished them. This means she went on to write the books, publish the books and market the books all as a single mother. Wow. That is amazing. Now I feel inspired.

20 March

I have been looking up baby names on the internet. Boys' names (to be completely honest) are actually quite boring.

We really want to find something different, a name that stands out but is easy to say, and a name that is easy to spell and doesn't rhyme with any swear words, body parts, or sexual positions.

So far we have thought of Bowie, yes, as in David Bowie, and Jude. We also like the name Neo *(from 'The Matrix' films)*. But we're not going to tell anyone our cool names.

21 March

A friend told us today that she knew a boy when she was little called Bowie. (Yes, we cracked under the pressure!) He lived down the street from her when she was young. She told us that Bowie used to eat the snot and boogas that hung out of his nose by licking them with his tongue. So instead of calling him Bowie, they called him BOGIE!!! Oh my god, I nearly barfed.

I guess we only have two names left now.

23 March

I have been trying not to swear so much. I've decided that good mothers don't swear. So I am not saying Fuck, or Cunt, Shit, or even Bloody anymore.

It's very difficult. It's almost like because I can't swear now I actually want to swear more. FUCK. See, I just need to get it all out - Fuck, Fuck, Fuck, Fuck, Fuck, Fuck, Fuck, Fuck, Fuck, Fuck, Fuck, Fuck, Fuck, Fuck, Fuck, Fuck, Fuck, Fuck.

There I think that's it... Oh, just one more...

Fuck!

WEEK 18

25 March

I went maternity shopping yesterday. Talk about expensive...! I had to give several blowjobs in the women's toilet just to pay for two garments. I knew it wouldn't be cheap, but I had to buy so many things. My stomach has just ballooned out in the last week or so and I am feeling like Humpty Dumpty.

Trying on maternity clothes was a slightly shocking revelation yesterday, as maternity clothes actually make you look *so* much more pregnant. (*Seriously - take Kylie Minogue, put her in some maternity gear, and she would look 56-months-gone.*) JC was shocked. I think reality set in yesterday when I came home and modelled my new fashion for him. He just couldn't believe it. "But you look so pregnant!" he said. (*What I think he wanted to say was; "But you look so fat!"*) I must admit though, these clothes are soooo comfortable and I feel much better wearing new maternity trousers instead of trying to squeeze into my old Diesel jeans.

Danni told me that her tummy started to show at about five months and said that because we were about the same size - bless her, I am so much fatter than she is - I would probably show around the same time. What I've learnt however, is that no two women are the same. I've been showing for two months now. I think my body decided from the start of this pregnancy that it was going to enjoy what it had been missing out on for so long…

A VACATION! With the banquet to match.

I have seriously been dieting for the last ten years of my life because of my work- and I mean strict dieting. I am not naturally thin. I have to work at it. So when I read at the start of my pregnancy that I should not diet, I was both petrified and overwhelmed with excitement at the same time.

So I have not been dieting. However, I am very thankful that I am not craving too many sweets. To be honest, I am not eating very much at all. Maybe it's because my uterus has expanded so much that my stomach is being squished up under my diaphragm and lungs fighting for space, and has therefore shrunk in size?

(OMG. Do I even know what I'm talking about?)

26 March

While shopping yesterday I was lucky enough to find a changing room with two mirrors - one for your tits and the other for your ass. I got a really good look at the second one…And oh my God, where do I start? Actually…There is no start. I couldn't tell where my thighs began and my ass ended. It has all melted together, and looks like one big giant bouncy castle. I am so depressed.

28 March

Yesterday we went for our first visit to the hospital, which was not at all what I expected. I had a vision of the hospital being really huge, like in American movies, painted white with pictures of bunny rabbits and giraffes on the maternity ward walls, doctors walking around chatting to each other in big oversized white coats.

Our hospital, however, is quite tiny and it's not even white. It's pale green, like a dentist's office.

Anyway, we tracked down a midwife that could speak English. Her name is Marie. We told her that we had chosen their hospital in which to have our baby. *(You can do this when you pay £400 a month for private insurance - thanks Starlight!)* Marie was really pleasant, informing me that I would need to give my details, have a check up *(probably to make sure I was pregnant instead of just being fat)* and have a consultation with a doctor, before we could be shown around the hospital.

The details: name, address, any previous illnesses, allergies, any ongoing medications, what my last surgical procedures were, if any.

I told her about the breast implants I had four years ago. Then *(quite hesitantly)* about the liposuction I had done two years ago. She then asked me on which part of my body I'd had it performed, to which I replied; "My stomach." I could see her laugh under her breath. "Yeah, ha ha." I bet she was thinking; "Fat good that bloody surgery is going to do you now!"

"OK that's fine," she concluded. "Now, let's have a look around."

I got very excited.

Marie showed us a delivery room first. It was quite big, and looked nothing like a hospital room at all. The bed for delivery was as big as our double mattress at home. There was also a birthing stool in there to squat on, a few machines and a lovely bay window overlooking the park *(which won't make any difference at all when I'm pushing Godzilla out of something the size of a ping pong ball).*

"Oh look at the beautiful park honey, there's some people feeding the ducks."

"Fuck off."

Marie said that if there were no complications, the baby would be delivered in here. (*Seemed like a good idea to me.)* The second room she showed us was a bit smaller. It only had a single bed (and a lot more machinery). She said this was the room that would be used if you needed an epidural. Obviously the bed was a lot smaller because you can't move around so much with a needle and tube stuck into your back. I decided I didn't really like this room as much. What I did like though were the two tiny newborn outfits laid out perfectly on a set of drawers next to me; one in pink and one in blue.

"Oh, how sweet - our baby gets to wear this little blue jumpsuit," I said to JC.

Then Marie proceeded to tell us that we didn't have to dress our baby in blue if we didn't want to, and it would be quite acceptable for our new born son to be dressed in pink if that's what we'd prefer? *(Yeah, OK!)*

Next Marie showed us the birthing pool, which I was quite surprised at because I thought only birthing centres had birthing pools. I was very excited. Adele has given birth twice in a pool, and has never torn at all. She says it's the best thing she ever did. (*Well, it would be wouldn't it - if your vag was still intact afterwards.)*

I told Marie that I wanted to have my baby in the pool. She laughed. She told me that even if you carefully plan your perfect labour, it never goes the way you think it will. In fact it almost always goes the opposite way entirely. I then proceeded to tell Marie that I loved pain, hated drugs and wanted to have my fanny split from the top of my clitoris down to my right ankle, and while being stitched up I wanted the nurse to take as long as possible so I could really experience the pain. *(Marie was not amused.)*

1 April

I am so excited! I have been feeling the baby move. It feels like butterflies are fluttering around inside me. It is so wonderful. I keep grabbing JC's hand and putting it on my belly. He says he can feel slight movements but I think he's lying to make me feel better. I guess I can feel it more intensely since it's coming from inside. Wow, I cannot tell you how amazing it is to feel the baby moving. It's as though there really is a little person inside you, funny that.

2 April

My boobs already have stretch marks on them, shit. My boobs have always been so beautiful and now they are ruined. I guess it doesn't help that I have a huge handful of silicone in each of them weighing them down. I fucking hate gravity. Obviously, that is why they are getting so big so quickly. I still have five months to go, not to mention the breastfeeding afterwards. I found out the other day that I might not even be able to breastfeed at all. There is a slight chance that I cannot. When the implants were put in, the incisions were made along the nipple line, so the milk ducts may have been severed. Apparently if the incisions are made underneath the breast or under the armpit breastfeeding is fine.

FUCK… How else am I going to lose all this weight?

3 April

I often wonder if other pregnant women are as full on as I am about pregnancy. I want to know everything there is to know- every symptom, every feeling, and every sensation. I have so many different kinds of books on pregnancy, and I am constantly searching on the Internet. I'm mad. I never even liked babies before. Now I'm obsessed. I think I am turning into a midwife. Soon I feel like I <u>will</u> know everything! Maybe I will be able to deliver my own baby?

4 April

I love being pregnant. I feel so fantastic all over, full of energy, and completely into it. We bought some baby clothes the other day, and they are just gorgeous, I just keep playing with them, fondling them, and pretending there's a baby inside.

Anyway, we went to see 'Coldplay' last night and they were fantastic. I even tried to go down the front and mosh out with JC *(just to be cool)*. However, I'm not cool. I'm pregnant. So after two minutes I went back up into the stalls and sat down to eat my ice cream.

5 April

Today some guys come around to fix the radiator in our bedroom. Boring.

They arrived at 9am in the morning (which is like 5am for show business folk). Too early! JC and I couldn't possibly keep sleeping in our bedroom while they hammered away, so we moved our mattress into the front room where we thought we would get a bit more sleep. After about 20 minutes, JC said; "Can you smell something burning?" He hesitated; "Oh my God, those guys are smoking in our bedroom!" I couldn't believe it. The nerve. JC got straight up and told the guys to put their cigarettes out because I was pregnant. I told him he should have told them to put their cigarettes out not only because I was pregnant, but because it was damn rude to smoke in a stranger's flat and where were they flicking their ash, anyway?

They really didn't think it was a big deal at all that I was pregnant. But of course **everything** is a big deal when you're pregnant.

7 April

Priscilla Presley… There you go. She was a young famous mum. She had Lisa Marie when she was just 23-years-old. And she's gone on to be successful. (*She was married to Elvis, which probably helped.*) If JC gets famous then I'm all set. Bring it on!

WEEK 19

8 April

I have been thinking about other pregnant women today, and how well they cope for nine months. Well it's actually ten months isn't it? I then started thinking about all the other mammals in the world, and wondered how long those mothers had to be pregnant for? I grew bored and began some research.

A dog pregnancy lasts 58 to 61 days.

A cat pregnancy lasts 60 to 65 days.

Oh… a giraffe pregnancy lasts 15 months.

Now I'm glad my neck is short!

9 April

I am sitting in the waiting room at Mrs Z's, waiting to be pricked and not looking forward to it.

JC and I went to Ikea this morning. We bought a brand new bed, it is soooo massive; I think it's the biggest one they sell. It's 180cm x 200cm and I love it. It has a beautiful big wooden base and two separate (German) mattresses, just in case I like to have my mattress hard and JC wants his soft - a pretty functional idea really. We had been sleeping on a much smaller mattress but I was getting too uncomfortable. For some reason I do not like JC touching me at all when we sleep now. He is really upset by this, but I told him it's not him, it's my hormones again; they're just so temperamental.

** Well, I just had my finger pricked *(not too bad this time)* and I've called JC so he can come in to watch the baby on the ultrasound and talk to Mrs Z. I am almost 20 weeks now, which means I'm half way there, yipeeeeeeeeeeeeeeeee eeeeeeee!

10 April

I have been so fussy lately, especially with my food! I want things to be exactly right or I won't even contemplate eating it. Today JC offered to make me some lunch. I said I wanted a few pieces of French stick with Vegemite and butter (which I was absolutely craving) but I only wanted the bread cut vertically, not horizontally, and I wanted the butter spread thinly, and the Vegemite just smeared across the top, NOT smudged into the butter. "Actually," I informed him, "just give me the knife and I will do it myself." He seemed rather upset, and proceeded to tell me that he feels absolutely useless lately because he cannot ever seem to do anything right for me. I said; "Babe, it's not you, it's me, and it's my body, my hormones." I explained; "My body is the court room and my hormones are the jury; evidence is then presented to the jury and they can dismiss or accept it. Even though I am the judge, the jury has the final say, and that's the verdict." JC thinks I'm a nutter.

12 April

That's it. I have given up wearing stilettos while I'm pregnant. It's official. I am now part of the flat shoe brigade, and I feel so normal, as normal as you can while looking like a baby hippopotamus. I knew the time would eventually come to take them off, and that time is now. I feel so unglamorous. It's pathetic.

14 April

Things have been a little difficult between JC and I at the moment. We have both been in tears the last few nights and I don't know what's going on. We have been arguing and are both so exhausted. It's all so messy.

Why are we fighting? I hate it. I can't stand it. I love him. I don't want to be fighting.

Subconsciously I know it's the baby. We are both afraid. But that's life. I hope things get better soon.

WEEK 20

15 April

Decided to go out tonight and see some friends play in their band. It was a cool night. Almost everyone from work came to the gig, so it was great to catch up with a few people (I have been confined to the house lately.) At one point, two friends of ours - Gavin and Elliot - were standing next to JC and I at the bar having a chat, when JC knocked Elliot's Jack Daniels out of his hand and the drink spilt all the way down the front of his new Versace shirt. JC was extremely apologetic.

Elliot replied; "Oh, don't worry about it, accidents happen!"

I pointed to my stomach and said; "I know."

Nobody laughed but me.

16 April

It's my birthday in three days and I've have decided to have a fancy dress party. Everyone has to dress up like a little kid, or in a kid's costume. And we are going to have children's games like pass the parcel, and an egg and spoon race. We have prizes to give away. We are making green cupcakes with purple icing, honey crackles, mini sausage rolls, party punch, and home-made Rocky Road. It's going to be great. We have even bought a little paddling pool to put out on our terrace, which will look amazing. And my fabulous friend Roberta is flying in from London and I am so excited to see her. Yeah!

17 April

The weather is so beautiful at the moment. It's almost too hot, I love it. I hope the weather stays like this for my 29th Birthday!

19 April

Happy Birthday Kelly

Woke up and had a glass of Möet. (*So shoot me.*) Who is going to arrest me? The pregnancy police? If I adhered to everything I read in those magazines and books, I would have to live in a cardboard box and only eat Weetabix.

Anyway, the party was so great. I dressed up as a fat little school girl, with a blonde curly wig and a pink dress with ribbons in my hair. JC dressed up as a French man. (He is a quarter French and looked very authentic.) We had a wonderful time. I especially enjoyed making a fairy castle cake from scratch. It was very pink and totally gorgeous. Then we all stuffed our faces, drank pink champagne (well I drank pink lemonade) and spent the day out in the sun getting drunk. It was a good birthday.

21 April

What a hideous day!! I woke up this morning feeling incredibly sick. I thought at first it was pregnancy-related but then JC told me he thought he was going to vomit, so he did. Then I said I thought I was going to vomit, so I did. And that was the start of our wonderful affair with the toilet. We both had gastroenteritis.

We must have puked and shat ourselves for at least 12 hours today. I was so worried to begin with, as all I could think about was the baby. However, after calling Mrs Z we were assured that the bug could not be passed on to the baby, and I was just going to have to go through it alone. I wasn't alone though. I had my wonderful husband to share the joy with. And I seriously cannot remember a time I have ever been that sick before. Nothing was making us feel better, nothing! We even watched 'Beaches', but that just seemed to make things worse.

What could have made us so ill? Was it the green cupcakes?

We found out later that everyone at the party got sick. Our friends' son came to my birthday yesterday when he was still a bit ill, and of course everyone who came into contact with him got sick, even his parents.

One thing today kept going over and over in my mind. "Imagine both of us being this sick in the future and having to look after the baby?" Actually I should re-phrase that. "There is definitely going to be a time in the future when we are going to have to go through that again, and look after the baby." Crap!

WEEK 21

22 April

I have woken up this morning and my tummy is really sore. It seems that my ligaments just keep stretching. The gastro, however, has gone. Thank God!

I talked to Adele today. I told her about my party and explained that I dressed up as a fat little school girl. She asked me why I didn't try Wonder Woman or Batgirl. I reminded her that Wonder Woman never got knocked up! I also told her that my stomach was way too big to hide, to which she replied; "How big can you be? You are only 18 weeks."

Firstly, I said; "I am not 18 weeks, I am 21 weeks." *(Because, of course, every week counts.)* "And secondly," I proceeded, "I am quite massive. I can't even see my fanny anymore."

"How many inches are you?" she asked. "Because when I gave birth to Noah, I was 43.3 inches around the largest part of my waist." I was so excited that I almost fell over my own feet leaping for the tape measure in the draw. I measured... 37.7 inches. Oh my God, 37.7. If I was 37.7 now, and I had 20 weeks left, how big was I going to get?

"37.7 inches," I told her. There was a slight pause.

"Oh poo," she replied. "Good luck with that."

25 April

As I was reading through a baby magazine today, I realised that I still do not have many of the second trimester discomforts that so many experts talk about.

I was so overjoyed in fact, that I decided to share the news with JC. "Guess what babe?" I said. "It says here that by now most women have experienced bleeding gums *(no)*, constipation *(no)*, haemorrhoids *(no)*, nasal discomfort *(no)*, pigmentation, no..." "Actually babe," he interrupted, "I forgot to tell you this the other day, but you do have some funny white spots on your face."

"What… Where?" I asked while running to the bathroom.

Then, looking into the mirror I saw them. Blotches. Fair, white blotches on my face.

"Bloody fucking unfair," I thought.

26 April

While reading a book by Dr. Miriam Stoppard today I flicked to the section dedicated to skin and hair care (which I found quite amusing). "With your eye make up, avoid hard colours as they will compete with the sparkle in your eyes." I laughed and thought; "Why not say? 'With your wardrobe, avoid any clothes, as they will compete with the bump on your stomach!'"

27 April

I have been feeling really horny lately. I want sex all the time. Luckily, so is my 20-year-old husband. We have been at it constantly lately and it's fabulous. I can't believe I want sex 4 or 5 times a day, it's insane…. Although JC says that's the way it should always be.

28 April

Today I went shopping and had to wee about a zillion times. The bathroom attendant in the toilets was asking 25c for each visit, and by the time it was 6pm I must have given him around 10 Euros. Next time I go back I think I will just ask for a four month pass.

Chapter 5

Gorillas in the Mist

"By far the most common craving of pregnant women is not to be pregnant."

Phyllis Diller

WEEK 22

29 April

My stomach won't stop hurting. I feel like I've eaten 12 meat pies, four bowls of carbonara and a stack of pancakes, washed down with two milkshakes. It's those damn ligaments stretching again. Or could it be gas? The thing is, if it is gas I don't want to sit on the toilet trying to do a poo because I've been told about haemorrhoids, and I don't want them. I've had them before, about three years ago. I had no idea what they were at the time, and I had no idea how I got them. My ass just really hurt. And it wasn't until I couldn't sit down anymore that I decided to take a look, and well… What can I say? My God! Those little buggers are just NASTY. Plus, they are in such an awkward place. After looking at them, your bloody neck hurts even more than your ass.

1 May

My belly is getting in the way of everything. It's constantly just THERE, 24-7. Everyday things are beginning to get hard. For instance, I can't even shave my legs anymore. It's too difficult - although I did a pretty good job yesterday, just took a deep breath, leant over my stomach and hacked away. I don't want to be a hairy Amazon you know. Already my minge has turned into a 'Gorillas in the Mist' sequel. Far out!

2 May

JC has a few days off so we have decided to go to Amsterdam. Yes, I know, it doesn't seem to be the most likely of destinations for a pregnant woman. However, Amsterdam is close, only two and a half hours on the train for us, and we thought it would be great to get away. It will be quite different compared to my last two visits because I won't be stoned this time.

5 May

Just returned from Amsterdam! We had such a great time…

We hired bikes and rode through the cobbled streets, and along the canals. I read somewhere that you shouldn't ride a bicycle after week 16 but I was absolutely fine and had no trouble, even though the pebbles in the road made me want to pee myself all the time. We went to a pancake restaurant and ate pancakes the size of cow patties. They were amazing. I love eating. I probably shouldn't but I can't help myself.

WEEK 23

6 May

I am so happy. I have dried up white goo on the inside of my bra… Is this colostrum? Adele seems to think so. She says I should have nothing to worry about now, as it looks like there is something passing through my nipples *(whatever it is)*.

I think I will most definitely be able to breastfeed. I am so relieved.

High fives all round to good plastic surgeons.

7 May

I measured my bits today. No! Not my vagina, but my body parts.

My new measurements are:

Waist - 36 inches

Hips - 38 inches

Bust - 39 inches

Thighs - 22 inches

8 May

I finally decided it was time to send an email home informing all my friends of my wonderful miracle of life.

The letter

Hi friends in Oz, Kelly here. Just thought I would be completely impersonal and send a group email, as I have not written for so long. You know...With all the drama in my life etc. The drama being that I am in fact pregnant, so my husband JC and I are going to have a baby (which a lot of you probably know already).

I know, I know, am I insane you ask? Yes, I believe I am. But I think it is one of the most fantastic decisions I have ever made. I am enjoying being pregnant. It is just such a blissful feeling, and I am looking forward to the challenge of motherhood; I mean don't get me wrong, I am also quite petrified. (I actually have poo running down my leg at this very moment.) But they say you should always welcome difficult challenges into your life with eager anticipation to experience who you really are and find out what kind of person you wish to become! (Who WAS that anyway? Gandhi?)

For those of you who never knew, I was in fact pregnant last year when JC and I came to Australia to get married in November, but on returning home here to Germany, I miscarried four hours after stepping through the front door. (Not extremely uplifting email material,

but nevertheless the truth about one of the unfortunate events in life.) I became pregnant again two weeks later. I guess Mother Nature obviously didn't want it any other way.

I never in my wildest dreams thought I would have a baby now. I mean I came over here to be a bloody star! However, I am very happy that I'm going to be a mum... and the feeling is something of complete and utter fulfilment that I guess only women can ever really truly experience (no offence guys). I really do have so much respect for mothers now; being pregnant is a hard job, considering the real job hasn't even started yet.

I have stopped working now, but the insurance company still pay me 90% of my wage until I am ready to go back to work, which will probably be three months after the baby is born (let's hope) so this makes circumstances very good. This way I can concentrate on the pregnancy while we save up money before we move to London where we plan to buy a house and live indefinitely.

I am now in my sixth month and due on 2 September, which seems forever away. I am enjoying being pregnant and at home everyday. I actually feel somewhat normal for a change. I'm also keeping journals of my pregnancy, and so far they are quite entertaining. So who knows, maybe I will write a book and get it published when I get to London. (Does anybody know how I would do that?)

So, with only three months to go I am getting quite nervous. My stomach is huge, absolutely enormous, because as you know my mother is a three foot pigmy, which makes me a towering five feet. Basically the only room for the baby to grow is OUT!

My belly measures 38.5 inches around the biggest part. (If you have a tape measure, go for it, it will really help you to appreciate your bodies like you never have before.) I have been feeling the baby move for about five weeks now, and man, is that weird or what! I feel like Sigourney Weaver with an alien living inside her. (Let's hope the baby that comes out isn't quite as ugly as that damn alien.)

One of the great things about being pregnant is the invisible Botox that has gone on within my skin. It's gorgeous, I look five years younger. I love it, and my hair, well… I should be in a fucking Pantene advert, it's fabulous…

Oh, did I mention that we found out the sex of the baby? We did, and we are having a boy! It's just so exciting, I think boys are fabulous. There will be no dealing with periods and boob jobs (just erections, wet dreams and masturbation.)

Anyway, I better go, however I hope everyone is wonderful, enjoying life, happy, and doing what they love…

I wish I had the time to write to each of you personally, however, I am usually too busy eating and weeing, so hopefully this email will suffice. Feel free to write whenever you have the time, it's always nice to receive an email from home.

I send each and every one of you my love and kisses, and hope to hear from you soon. Keep happy (and keep your legs together girls).

All my love Kel xxx

9 May

I need to wax my damn bikini line, but I can't see it. I am going to need some help, but frankly I don't know if I can trust JC. I know he will want to take it all off, and probably rip off a piece of my labia in the process. However, that hair needs to go.

10 May

A friend of a friend told me today that her friend's mother used to smoke dope everyday whilst she was pregnant! This makes me feel better, as lately I have been feeling somewhat concerned about the pot I smoked five months ago.

I told Mrs Z about it the other day, and she said that a lot of people drink and smoke before they realise they are pregnant, but it rarely makes any difference, except in extreme cases of addiction. However, JC and I are a bit worried. We want our baby to be so perfect. Hearing this story today puts my mind at ease a little. I mean, if this woman was smoking pot everyday, and her daughter turned out to be fine, well, then I guess there is hope left for the rest of us.

11 May

I am going to count how many times I wee today because, well, basically I've got too much time on my hands. It is 12:24pm now, and so far I've peed six times since I got up at 7:30am. I am almost convinced that I pee every hour, so I guess we will wait and see.

OK, it's now 11pm and I have gone for 19 wees so far, and to be completely honest I just cannot be bothered counting anymore.

12 May

I have been meditating quite a bit lately and I feel really great. It is quite hard to get into it sometimes, but it really works. I am such a big thinker, always planning, devising, doing, going, creating. My mind races so fast, so meditating really works for me. I feel as though it puts all the jigsaw pieces together that are usually randomly floating around my head. I just try to concentrate on my breathing, and nothing else.

I also have a great book called 'A Joyful Birth – a Spiritual Path to Motherhood'.

Compiled by Susan Piver, it's so cute and one of the most amazing books I've read. There are so many different elements to this book.

The first chapter is absolutely incredible, written by a woman called Anne Cushman, a yoga teacher. She writes about being pregnant, giving birth and becoming a mother, which is really incredible and will stay with me for as long as I can remember.

Several other women also write in this little book about the fears of motherhood (and birth) bonding with your baby, and looking after and nourishing yourself as well. There are aromatherapy treatments and diagrams of yoga positions for pregnancy, and also some fantastic meditations included, complete with two CDs which contain meditation for mother and baby and just some overall relaxation music for mum. I love the CDs, they take me away.…. And the meditations are great, just 10 minutes each and fantastic. They are perfect for deep relaxation, and a woman with a lovely voice talks you through the meditation which I find perfect. The women who write in this book are so inspirational. What they have to say is brilliant and real, and authentic.

This book is amazing.

WEEK 24

14 May

I feel fantastic today. I think it's all the sex I've been having. My hormones feel as though they are on holiday in Ibiza. I am feeling like some kind of primitive beast. However sex is becoming more difficult. It's hard for JC to lie on top of me anymore as he squashes my tummy when he gets too excited, so I usually lay on him, although I feel like a fat warthog.

We have tried a few different positions, like JC sitting on the edge of the bed while I straddle him, but last time we did that I fell onto the floor and hit my head on the wardrobe.

I was just too heavy. I weigh more than JC now, so how is he supposed to support me?

Oral sex though is absolutely brilliant. And a quote from one of my best friends PJ comes to mind here when I say; "Get down there and don't come up until your face turns blue."

15 May

My tummy is hurting a bit this morning. I think it's because it's stretching. I also have haemorrhoids, ouch. I feel so fragile.

I am getting my hair done today, having some streaks put in. Some books say this is bad for baby, but it would be worse for mother to have ugly hair and be depressed.

16 May

I could hardly sleep last night, I was so uncomfortable, and I had itchy legs again. I tried lying on my back with my legs up on the wall at one point, but it didn't really help. I'm guessing that my legs aren't getting proper circulation (probably due to all the new fat cells) and that's why they itch and feel heavy. JC massages them for me sometimes, but I didn't want to ask him to do it for me last night because I feel like I am always asking him to massage something…

I found a solution to my problem last night when all else failed. (*Well it worked last night, and if it doesn't work again I'm going to have to have an affair with a masseur.*) I pop myself into an empty bath, take an exfoliator and some soap and vigorously massage my legs, from top to bottom, then I rinse them off with extremely cold water. The feeling of weightlessness in my legs afterwards is pure heaven.

17 May

I was standing in front of the oven today; baking a cake, when the little man kicked me really hard about three times. After I looked down, I realised my belly was really hot and I had been resting it on the front door of the oven. Fuck, I didn't even feel it because the skin has obviously stretched so far now, the nerves are numb.

Poor little tiger, he was getting cooked in there. I was making baby cakes.

18 May

I decided yesterday that I would get away for a few days and come and stay with some friends of JC's family - Sue and Michael. They live in a town called Fockinghausen. (Yes, it makes me laugh every time I hear it.) JC has been working so hard, and I have been babbling on and on about baby shit for so long, we are both a bit sick of each other and there seems to be a lot of tension around the house at the moment.

So I caught the train for an hour tonight - quite an ordeal. I hadn't reserved a seat for myself, so I just sat down where I wanted, only to be kicked off the seat 10 minutes later by someone who HAD reserved a seat.

Anyway, with one big bag and one big belly I waddled down several carriages looking for a seat. The conductor saw that I needed help and found me a seat next to a 50 year old dirty man who smoked like a chimney, so I moved again (*not wanting baby to be born with emphysema*). I was so tired by this point and I just wanted a seat. After 10 minutes of searching I walked past a group of young guys who were blocking the aisles with their luggage and their beer breath. They didn't offer to move their bags at all and as I walked past them instead of asking them to help me I just burst into tears. *(They moved their luggage after this, but - Bloody Hell!)* I was so upset, nothing was going smoothly and I ended up sitting on my piles on the floor of the train looking like a pilgrim.

19 May

Sue and Michael's house is wonderful. They live near a big forest that belongs to a Duke, so I go walking through the woods in the morning. I even started singing today. I haven't really sung in ages. Just as I set out I saw a deer. It had stopped in its tracks and was listening to me. I felt like Snow Fucking White. It was brilliant. It's really nice to be by myself. I am really relaxed here. It's quiet and my mind and body get to rest. It's what I needed really. I don't have any house work to do, or any responsibilities and I get somebody else cooking for me every night. I am loving it.

WEEK 25

20 May

I popped on Sue's scales today, and I weigh 10.18 stone. Oh my God, the last time we were here at Christmas I weighed 8.3 stone. I have put on almost 26.4 pounds already, and I just finished eating four pieces of toast, so no doubt that has added a bit extra on. Shit!

In the book 'Mother and Baby Care' the model has put on eight pounds to date. What does she eat? Folic acid? This is totally unfair. I look at these books as a source of constant comfort. Does every woman who reads these books feel inadequate? Or am I the only woman who is putting on enough weight to feed the whole of South East Asia?

I think it's time someone published a book that shows real life women, women who don't always look glamorous in gorgeous maternity wear because in real life they can't actually find anything to wear.

Women who aren't smiling like a toothpaste advert because their haemorrhoids are so uncomfortable they haven't been able to do a shit for five days.

Women who don't always have their hands clasped gently over their beautiful full pregnant bellies because, let's face it, their hands are too busy trying to strangle the partners who got them into the mess in the first place.

Also - why do all the women's husbands in these books look so damn serious all the time? Are they all bankers? Why can't they show photos of men smiling, looking as though they are excited about the birth of their child? Not as though all they're thinking is; "How much do nurseries cost?"

And why are they never good looking? I would have never wanted a child if my partner had a high forehead and a long moustache.

21 May

Sleeping comfortably has now become a thing of the past. Goodbye sleep. It was fun while it lasted. There are only two positions I can actually sleep in now: on my right side with a pillow between my knees and on my left side with a pillow between my knees. (*Sometimes, if I really treat myself, I place two pillows between my knees.*)

It's not fair. I thought maybe in the last couple of months I would be sleep deprived, but not <u>now</u>... The last five nights have been a nightmare.

I'm on my way home now and have an appointment at 11:30am with Dr Z. I am soooooo looking forward to seeing our son on the big screen again. It has been six weeks since we saw the sequel to his debut movie 'Dancing with my Placenta' and I am so excited!

Adele said I should feel very privileged to see our baby on the ultrasound quite so much because she only ever has two ultrasound checks in Oz, one at 19 weeks and one at 30 weeks. I actually love that bloody ultrasound so much that I want to go out and buy one myself, so I can see the little man everyday. How much do you think they cost?

22 May

I have just finished reading 'Have the birth you want' by Gill Thorn.

This book was really great and extremely informative. I liked how it started with a brief history of birth. It was amazing to read about women 50 years ago and what they had to go through. Gill even goes back to the 1500's and tells how midwives who tried to relieve a mother's pain with particular remedies were thought to be witches and burnt at the stake. She then goes on to explain how maternity care has improved over hundreds of years. Today women are able to give birth in a safer environment than ever before.

The title does not really match the contents however. Gill is very pro natural birth, and the whole way through the book she explains why a natural birth is better and how she thinks technology is introduced into women's labours these days when it is not really necessary. This is a good point, but I am not personally so focussed on having a natural, active birth. I mean, I would like too but if my body feels like it's being torn in two, I will not hesitate to scream; "Fuck natural birth, give me an epidural now!" Gill made me feel slightly guilty about wanting drugs (how dare she!) I believe it's important to have the birth you want, but I do not want to be in so much pain that I cannot enjoy it. I want to be present, I want to be comfortable. I can put up with pain, but I think Gill should give equal weight to both sides of the debate. Still, I could not put the book down. She covers everything in extreme detail. I especially like what she writes about the risks in pregnancy and how she puts them into perspective, because I think every mother is concerned about the well-being of her unborn child.

Gill expresses it perfectly; "Nobody really expects to be the one in a million who wins the dream holiday in a prize draw but being the one whose baby has a problem seems frighteningly possible." Yep, she hit it on the head there!

Overall, this is a wonderful book and I found myself reading it over and over again. It gave me a sense of confidence as Gill writes with great optimism and enthusiasm. She makes you feel as though you are completely in control of how you want to deal with your own pain and the overall perception of fear.

Thanks Gill, you're a gem.

23 May

I went for my 25 week check up yesterday and everything is OK. I was in there for about two hours (which totally sucked and is quite boring when all you have to read is a German copy of 'Cosmopolitan'.) The fact that I got to see our little man on the screen was sufficient compensation. It was great. The full blown blood test I had was not so great and Mrs Z found traces of blood in my urine. OUCH! She said it was not coming from my vag but from my bladder and that it may be caused by the baby rubbing on it. OUCH again! She said I may also have a small infection. She told me to drink copious amounts of water and report back to her immediately if I have any kidney or abdominal pain. She also said a urinary tract infection would not be good right now, as it could lead to premature labour if not diagnosed and treated early on. Shit!!

I have therefore been drinking so much water I feel like a whale. *(Do whales drink water?)*

24 May

I am so forgetful lately. I walked all the way to the DVD shop today, only to forget the DVDs I was supposed to return. Fuck, fuck, fuck. It was a good fifteen minute walk there, and fifteen minutes back, but not something that I would like to do twice in one day. I know it's probably good exercise, and I need to be as fit as I can for the birth, but I really can't be buggered today. Isn't pregnancy hard enough without having to walk?

26 May

Since JC missed out on the last visit, we decided that we would go back to Mrs Z today so he could see the baby. I was only in there four days ago, so I was actually feeling a bit weird asking for another ultrasound; however Mrs Z was only too happy to oblige…

JC was really amazed at how big our boy looked, and yes, he is definitely a boy. I saw a huge ball bag in there. (*I actually thought it was his head, and his legs were his arms.*) He looked so beautiful and I must admit that I just fall more deeply in love with him every time I see him. He was moving around a lot, looking like he was doing water aerobics. I guess he has a lot of room in there. JC also noticed that when Mrs Z placed the ultrasound thingy on my tummy, the little man turned his head right toward the camera!

He's obviously going to be an actor.

Chapter 6

Cellulite knees

*"Stressed spelled backwards is desserts. Coincidence?
I think not!"*

Anonymous

WEEK 26

27 May

Had a massive fight with JC last night. It was awful.
I know I am a bit mad and psychotic at the moment due to
the stretching of my stomach but no one should piss off a
pregnant woman. In 'Becoming a Mother' Kate Mosse says
the Hittites, who ruled Babylon from 1600 to 1200 BC (*yes,
I had to look that up*), were forced 'to pay 10 shekels of silver
for inflicting actual or emotional harm on a woman in the
later stages of pregnancy, (but) only five shekels if she had not
passed her sixth moon month'.

Well, what about today? I don't know how much a
shekel might be worth now but five must be enough to buy

myself a good vibrator and get rid of my husband for a few days, surely?

28 May

That's it, I can't walk anymore, everything hurts and it's not fair. I've always walked everywhere, but now after only one hour I am in complete pain. It's my feet. They are just so sore - the balls, the heels, the toes, the hair on my toes, the lot. I think it's the heaviness of my fat ass!

I'm sick of being fat today. I desperately want a day off. I want to peel all the excess fat off my body and give it to a butcher.

While I'm at it, I'd like to give this bump to my husband, so he can feel how utterly annoying it is. Yes, just for a day so I could put on my bikini, lay out in the sun, drink a Long Island Iced Tea, eat brie and pate, have runny eggs on toast, smoke a big fat joint and look down and see my little minge again. Ahh, sounds like bliss.

29 May

It's taking too long, I've had enough, I don't want to play anymore. I've been pregnant for a good six months now. It's not even nine months you're pregnant for anyway - it's 10, and that is false advertising!

However, we did get a new pushchair today from some friends of some friends. Well… it's actually far from new, but nevertheless it is a pushchair, a very cheap pushchair. The only thing is… that… well… it's ugly.

It was designed in the 80's, and it looks, well, how can I say it? Naff. Both JC and I are thankful for the discounted second hand pushchair; however we are both quite disappointed that we don't get to go shopping to look for a new one ourselves. It's fun to look around baby stores when you're expecting a baby. I think for mothers it's even more exciting than oral sex! We also wanted a pushchair that was trendy and cool; I mean, we are young, hip parents. Danni and Matt came around today and said it was great. They also said that even if you buy a new pushchair, it ends up looking crap in a few months anyway; and at least we were saving some cash. This is true, because they are expensive. Advertisers put big bucks into selling baby stuff and we won't fall for it. Maybe our pushchair is OK? I guess it has saved us money, money we can spend on something else, like ourselves! It's not all about the baby you know. I mean, we've still got to look good, don't we?

1 June

Over the weekend I went to see JC in Starlight. Just before I walked into the theatre a woman called Beergit (*pronounced Beer Gut*), who works there and has children of her own, said to me; "Oh, are you sure your baby will be OK with the loud music? He might be frightened." She then told me that when she was pregnant with her last child, she went to see Lethal Weapon 4 and her baby just squirmed and squirmed because he hated the loud noises in the film; it scared him.

I said; "My baby doesn't get scared, he's a soldier."

2 June

I sat down on the couch last night and suddenly realised while looking down at my knees, that I have cellulite on them! How can I have cellulite on my knees? It's bad enough having it on my butt, but my butt I can hide. I can't hide cellulite knees - not in summer. I showed JC and he just laughed, and assured me that you couldn't really notice them. I think it's all the cookies I've been eating. I've been really into baking cookies lately and really into eating them as well. Cookie knees, that's what I have. OK. No more cookies. I should really be eating fruit and vegetables, or maybe I should bake fruit pies, or apple crumble, then I wouldn't feel so guilty.

WEEK 27

4 June

A Poem

I woke up this morning and realised that I'm actually having a baby.

This bump on my front isn't full of cream buns; I'm a very pregnant lady.

It just seems so weird that I am changing; I cannot believe he's inside,

A fully formed baby with a teeny tiny body, a sweet little mouth and two eyes.

I often wonder what he'll look like? Will he look anything like me?

Will he be gorgeous, clever, funny, or short
(because I'm only four foot three)?

And I wonder if the baby hears when I sing and
talk and dance?

Does he know when I think of giving birth that I
want to poo my pants?

Will the labour be painful? And how will it start?
I really can't help but think?

Will I be doing the shopping, watching the telly, or
standing by the sink?

And when he comes home, just what will we do?
When does he sleep and feed?

Do I become his maid - running, tits out, to meet
his every need?

Will I tear out my hair because he cries all day?
Will I get the baby blues?

Will I even be able to wee cos my fanny will be so
bruised?

And when will I be able to make love to my man?
When can he pop it in?

Will my figure ever come back...?   When will I
be thin?

I think and I wait, I dream and I pray; "Please
God make it go fast."

And while you're there just one more thing;
"Please take this fat off my ass!"

5 June

Well, a whole load of books arrived for me today so I am rather excited. I ordered them from Amazon. I was particularly looking forward to 'Prenatal Pregnancy', a spiritual guide to loving your unborn child. I have already read about 12 books on pregnancy, most of them to do with women's changing bodies, changing attitudes, what to expect in your first year, common pregnancy complaints and other women's birth stories etc. However I have been really interested in finding out how to form a special bond with your baby while he's in the womb, and this book is all about that. I am so hip!

6 June

Our first baby was due today. That feels a bit weird. I could not imagine having another baby other than this little man inside me now. Still I am a bit sad as I keep thinking about how hard it was when I miscarried seven months ago.

It was so terrible. Nevertheless, it makes me really appreciate what I have now.

7 June

Last night was so hot. I need to have the small fan on blowing wind at my face; otherwise I cannot get to sleep at all. It's getting to that stage now where I am beginning to feel uncomfortable. I thought that maybe I could be superwoman and transcend all those common third trimester discomforts, however I can see that I may be wrong.

So far my pregnancy has been fabulous, minus those first three months of morning sickness. I hate damn morning sickness.

And anyway, why is it that women get morning sickness but all men get is bloody morning glory?

WEEK 28

10 June

I've worked out that I can officially walk for one hour a day before my feet feel like they are about to burst like fat balloons. I love walking *(just about as much as I love sleeping)* but is there not ANYTHING I can do normally anymore? I have started to develop a distinct waddle, so my walking is somewhat handicapped. Instead of moving in a straight line, I sway from side to side like a metronome. My legs are also rubbing together from the top of my thighs down to the bottom of my knees. *(If they were two pieces of wood I could start a fire.)* The thing is, I feel great, I have energy, I love this pregnancy business, but I can now see why Adele laughed after I told her that the next three months were going to fly past. The days are getting longer. I still have 83 days to go, WOW, that's 83 sleeps! That means if I'm weeing 19 times a day, that's 1577 more times I have to piss before the baby comes out.

11 June

Last night I got JC to trim my pubic hair for me, which was an extremely scary procedure as I couldn't see what he was doing at all. 'The bump' is just too big. Letting someone trim your bush is all about trust, a bit like that game you play at school where someone stands behind you, you close your eyes, and then fall backwards and let them catch you. If the person behind you doesn't catch you, you will fall and hit the ground. If you let someone cut your pubic hair with large kitchen scissors, one wrong snip could leave you clitoris-less. *(I can understand why they don't play this game at school.)*

Fortunately for me, JC did a good job, and now I have a neat, trim, and extremely <u>itchy</u> vagina, even if I can't see it.

12 June

I have just been reading 'Prenatal Parenting' by Frederick Wirth. It's very interesting (although quite full on and very intense.)

Frederick is very passionate about what he writes and believes from his own studies (and the studies of others) that as a mother you have influence over your unborn baby's brain architecture, which will affect your child for the rest of its life.

"This exploration actually starts twelve weeks prior to birth and continues until the child reaches his second birthday…These experiences during these important twenty-seven months actually shape the architecture and biochemistry of his developing brain."

See, told you it was quite full on…

Frederick believes that the thoughts we think and the actions and reactions we have in life while we are pregnant effect the foetus in the womb directly by messenger molecules known as Neuro-peptides, which pass through the blood stream and cross the placenta. "Inside the womb, the infant directly experiences his mother's external circumstances."

"You and your unborn infant are connected in a most intimate way by the passage of Neuro-peptides across the placenta. These powerful molecules affect your unborn child's prenatal emotional development by altering brain structure." Woah!!!!!!

So if I masturbate a lot, and think dirty thoughts, will my baby grow up to be a pervert?

Basically, he's saying that the way we act and the responses we have to certain situations will affect our baby forever.

"A child's personality is in place long before he enters preschool. Psychologists tell us they can recognize which children are going to get into trouble in their teenage years by the time they are two years old."

He also talks about self esteem, working through your fears, assessing and changing negative behaviours, and of course how to communicate directly with your unborn child through reading, singing and taking what he calls 'foetal love breaks'.

You can tell he is American, but if you want a challenge and something interesting to do while you're pregnant (and you are unemployed) this is a great book.

13 June

I am getting very emotional about people not noticing that I'm pregnant, and just treating me like a normal person. I was standing in line at H&M today when, after waiting at the front of the line for what seemed like 20 minutes, three young girls walked straight past me and waltzed into the very cubicle that I had just been waiting for. Now... I've never wanted to get aggressive with anyone in public before, but this time I was fucking furious!

I was so sore and tired and just wanted to get home and rest. But these girls completely pissed me off. I wanted to yell; "Hey, wait a minute, I was next." But my brain didn't work that fast, so I didn't say anything. Instead I waited, waited until I could prepare myself before attempting to speak my very best German to them. *(N.B. I didn't prepare myself very well, and proceeded to talk to them in my very finest English instead.)*

"Hey girls," I said finally when they emerged from the cubicle giggling. "Firstly, I'm really sorry I have to speak to you in English." *(I wasn't sorry at all.)* "But my German is not good enough to find all the rude words I'm about to say to you." They looked puzzled. I went on. "I don't think I have ever seen such complete and utter ignorance in my whole life." They stared at me and I could see they were trying their best to understand. "I was actually waiting at the front of the line when you all so rudely pushed right in front of me. Now as you can probably see, I'm pregnant. I realise you have no idea what being pregnant feels like. It's a tough business. Your feet ache, along with your back, you get fat and things hurt. Now the last thing you want to be doing is waiting in a queue for 20 minutes for a change room, when three 15 year old pimple-faced girls fuck you over by pushing in front of you." They were silent. I continued; "Furthermore, it was not only me you were pushing in front of, but 10 other ladies behind me… You dumb little whores!"

Well…

That's what I would have liked to say. Truth is, I didn't say anything at all. I just gave them a smile, paid for my new skirt and went on my way.

14 June

I can't breathe. I mean, of course I can breathe, but I only ever take short shallow breaths these days. I just want to be able to breathe normally.

JC cut himself with a kitchen knife this morning. There was blood everywhere and I couldn't bear it. Usually I am fine with blood and have a high tolerance to gore, but this morning...No way! I just couldn't stomach it. How am I going to deal with child birth? One look at the blood on the kitchen floor this morning and I was ready to pass out.

Anyhow, I rang the director from the show straight away and told him JC wouldn't be coming in because he'd butchered himself and we took him to the hospital, where we waited for four hours to see a doctor.

15 June

JC and I suddenly decided last night that we wanted to go to London. So we did. I love being spontaneous! We were both sitting on the couch looking at a copy of English 'Vogue', admiring the fashion, when JC said; "I wish we could go shopping in London instead of this crappy town." I replied; "Well, why don't we go? You have a few days off, we could leave tomorrow morning and be back on Tuesday."

WELL... Talk about excitement, we were both beaming, and felt like little kids going to Disneyland. So we got on the net, booked two tickets, and within seven hours we were on a plane. How easy was that? However, at 28 weeks, I was supposed to have a letter from my doctor stating that I was healthy, there were no complications with my pregnancy and I was OK to fly. However I couldn't get a letter, it was Sunday, and I wanted to go to London! I decided that if anyone at the airline asked, I would tell them I was only 27 weeks. But no one even noticed I was pregnant. The woman checking in our luggage even asked if I wanted the window seat. Which of course I didn't! I wanted the isle seat for easy access to the toilet. Bitch!

Anyhow, the flight was great, and we were feeling high and free. Then I wondered whether a trip like this would have been so spontaneous and possible with a baby? I mean how much different would it be? We would have to take the baby of course, a Moses basket for the baby to sleep in, clothes for the baby, a pushchair, baby blankets, nappies, a baby bag to carry all of baby's things, bottles (for other people to feed the baby since I would want to shop in London- which also means I would have to take my express pump), and I think that's it really. Oh hang on - some soft towels for baby, baby wipes, diaper cream, breast pads, thermometer, dummies, bottle warmer, baby's passport, holy shit. OK. I can kind of understand now why parents go on about a baby changing your life sooooo much.

It still sounds like fun to me.

A friend of a friend told me once that 'you don't fit into the baby's life, the baby fits into yours.' This woman was an entertainer, who would take her son with her to every job; she would just organise to have a nanny supplied by the company she was working for. She took her baby to Greece,

America, France and Spain; actually come to think about it, that woman may have been Victoria Beckham.

16 June

London is fabulous and today we went shopping in Covent Garden. JC was determined to buy some funky clothes, and I was determined this time to find Mothercare. And luckily I did, oh yes, I did. And it was like having an orgasm for the very first time. I never realised going to a major baby store could be quite so exhilarating. I was in heaven. I spent over an hour and a half in there, and could have gone completely mad. A mother's dream. There were so many cute baby clothes in there, just gorgeous, outfits of Tigger and Winnie the Pooh, tiny jackets and booties and hats, and great maternity wear. I bought myself a dress, which fits my bump sensationally, and I actually feel glamorous in it. Downstairs there was furniture, push chairs, changing tables, high chairs, books, toys and lots of mothers and babies. It was so wonderful, I had the greatest time.

WEEK 29

17 June

Just got back from London. My parents called me today and said that they had received the photos of me pregnant, and while dad told me I looked wonderful I could hear mum in the background shouting; "Your arms are a bit fat", to which I replied; "Yes, thank you for telling me, cause we don't have a mirror at home." My dad was sweet though. He said; "You're pregnant, you're allowed to have chubby arms." So, that was a real boost to my confidence. I mean I know that I look a bit chunkier, but when other people point it out, well, that's just too much of a reality check. I even rang Adele afterwards to get a second opinion, as she also had the photos. Without hinting I said; "So did you like the photos?" She quickly replied; "You look like me when you're pregnant; you get fat arms too… I call myself Beefcake Baillie when I'm pregnant." *(Baillie is her married name).* "So what shall I call myself?" I thought. "Obese O'Brien?" Or maybe I should just call myself 'Big fat frumpy cow who has no self control because she doesn't exercise enough and has been eating cookies and cream buns almost everyday and will have to join Weight Watchers as soon as she's finished breast feeding O'Brien?'

20 June

I love to lie down and watch my tummy move; it's the most amazing thing. I could do it for hours. I try to guess where the little man's body parts are in relation to my tummy. I think it makes him feel more real to me to see him move about. I still can't believe sometimes that there's actually a baby in there. I wish women's stomachs were like glass, and then you could just look at them all the time. Then again, maybe not- that would be quite gross come to think of it. *(Do I just talk for the sake of it?)*

21 June

I called Adele today and asked her if she could tell me all three of her birth stories. She said she didn't have a spare 24 hours, but she could tell me about the birth of her first-born, her daughter Jazmyn.

ADELE'S BIRTH STORY GOES LIKE THIS

With Jazmyn I had an appointment when I was one week overdue, it was a Tuesday. I was already freaking out because I was only 21 at the time, it was my first baby and I didn't really know what to expect. I had chosen to go to a birthing centre, about 45 minutes away from home because I wanted to have a natural birth. When I arrived at my appointment the midwives told me that the baby was fine (though not ready to emerge yet) and assured me that the baby would probably come any day now. To me it seemed as if they didn't really care, they were just so nonchalant about the whole thing, which really got to me at the time. Looking back I guess they were all very experienced, and used to this kind of thing... It was me who was the amateur! Anyway, I left without making another appointment, since I would be giving birth 'any day now'. Four days later on the Saturday, the midwife called and asked me if I wanted to come in. She said; "We'll see if we can do something?" I was a bit anxious as I didn't really know what the midwives were going to do. However I told my husband Matt that we were going in to the birthing centre tomorrow so they could 'do something' to me, having absolutely no idea what they were going to do? (*N.B. My sister Adele is now a midwife.*) So we went in on Sunday morning about 11am with my bags packed. First thing they did when we got there was give me an internal, and whilst the midwife put her fingers up my nooni, she proceeded to give me some very explicit audio/

visual commentary, explaining that my cervix was like a bag of marbles with a draw string attached to the top. If the marble bag was a bit loose then she could unplug the mucus plug, known as a show *(yes Adele, I know)* and start the labour. I was quite uncomfortable by this stage, not only physically but also by someone referring to my cervix as a bag of marbles. As it happened, the marble bag was loose and she was able to take the plug out. She then told me I might start having contractions a little bit later in the day, although I was expecting to go into labour more or less straight away. Then they sent me home.

At about 2:30pm the same day I started having contractions about every three minutes; they didn't really hurt that much, and I just lay on the couch breathing while Matt fixed the roof outside, since we had just moved into our new house. I kept breathing through my contractions for several hours; we even went to church that night where I kept timing my contractions (still three minutes apart.) By the time we got home though the contractions were a lot more intense. So we got into the car and drove to the birth centre. I figured they would probably just send me home again because I didn't know whether my contractions were intense enough. However, when we got there they told me to stay since I was already 12 days overdue. This really helped to relax me and ease my mind because I didn't want to go home again. The birth centre was great because they had a television and a VCR there (which helped take my mind off the most intense pain I was ever going to experience in my life). An hour later they gave me another internal. "OK... well you're three centimetres dilated so that's great news". I was like; "Yeah, woo hoo". By this stage my contractions felt like really awful period pain, and I was having to concentrate and breathe through them so I could cope with the pain. I tried moving around at one stage but that only made the pain worse, so we sat down and watched movies, although I kept grunting every three minutes for about 30 seconds to get through the contractions.

This went on all through the night. Matt and I watched two movies and went for a few small walks, but by 5am I said that I wanted another internal to see how dilated I was. To my surprise I was still three centimetres, and I felt like I wanted to punch the midwife on the nose. I had been three centimetres for 15 hours. I said; "You're joking, I've been in all this discomfort and agony for hours, and nothing's happened?" She said; "Well, I can break your waters for you if you like?" "OK," I replied, even though I was a little bit apprehensive about this. So she broke my waters and all of a sudden I was in complete and utter pain, it hurt so much. I felt like I wanted her to put all the water back in so the pain would go away. It was awful. I was just in so much pain and immediately I could feel this big head pushing against my butt. I thought; "Oh my goodness, I'm gonna poo myself." So I raced for the loo. Now, I thought it hurt before, but whilst on the toilet I truly felt like I was going to die. I was sitting there for ages, then started yelling; "It's coming, it's coming." It hurt so much. The midwife then told me to stick my finger up there to see if I could feel the head. I thought; "Are you serious? And are you allowed to do that? It sounds a bit freaky to me." Anyway, I did, and right at the end of my finger I could feel this really hard bit, and hair! I almost passed out; it was the weirdest sensation, just so bizarre. I thought; "Far out! There's someone inside me!"

I then decided to get into the spa which felt great, but all of a sudden I was just so thirsty because it was so hot and I was obviously dehydrated. So in between contractions I was drinking litres and litres of water. Then the pain got worse, and I thought I was really going to explode. I sat up on my hands and knees, holding on to a pole at the back of the spa, then Matt came around to me so I could concentrate and focus on him. The pain was terrible. Then I leaned up against Matt and bit into his arm really hard, I didn't realise that I was doing it at the time, and he had a big bite mark there later. I needed some gas. However my midwife was this old Scottish lady who made me feel absolutely terrible when I asked for some. She was not only peeved that I wanted it, but also that she had to go and get it. She made me feel so awful, not that she said anything, but that she just seemed reluctant to help, which made the whole scenario even worse. She eventually got it and it was so great, as it gave me something to concentrate on. I was only supposed to breathe the gas in when I was having contractions but I kept sneaking breaths when Mrs McGregor wasn't looking. She kept catching me though, saying; "Stop breathing it in." I couldn't believe it, she was telling me off! I could have strangled her. I thought; "I can't do this anymore." I really thought I was going to pass out, but the midwife reassured me that I was nearly there.

Right about then Mrs Grumpy McGregor's shift was up and another midwife came on duty - Julie my favourite midwife. It made me so happy to see her I almost cried. Julie was fantastic. She was positive, encouraging and like a breath of fresh air. I kept asking Julie; "How much longer, How much longer?" All she kept saying was; "Not long, not long."

Just then the phone rang, I was so angry, it was just too much, it made everything so realistic. I hated it. I thought my head was going to spin around and around and I was going to explode, I was about to erupt with violent anger, and I realised that Matt and I had given the phone number out to both of our parents and they were the ones who were probably calling. (It was Matt's mother.) Fortunately the phone rang out and I could concentrate on Matt again, who just had this horrible worried look in his eyes, he had no idea what to do, he looked so stressed and freaked out; he wanted to help me but he didn't really know how. The funny thing was that he knew he was supposed to keep telling me how wonderfully I was doing, and he was, but his face was completely contradicting his words, so it wasn't really very reassuring. Then it was time. Julie said; "OK Adele, do you feel like pushing?" I thought; "NO." Then about two seconds later I got this massive urge to push, a very strange feeling of wanting to do the biggest poo. It was so weird thinking that there was something in there. I just wanted to get it out. I could really feel the head creeping down and couldn't do anything to stop it. It was such a strange sensation (as well as downright painful) and I didn't want the head to come out, but I couldn't do anything to stop it. Then out it came. All I kept thinking to myself was; "I can't believe I am doing this? I can't believe this is me giving birth right now." It all seemed like an out of body experience. Then Julie said "OK, come on… Just one more push and the baby will be out." And as much as I wanted the baby to be out, I really didn't want to push. I didn't want to go through anymore pain. I thought; "Just leave the baby in there like that, and I will walk around the rest of my life with a baby's head sticking out in between my legs." However, the next contraction came, and I couldn't help but push the rest of the baby out. I was so exhausted. I thought; "Finally, it's all over." Then I put my head down on my chest and let out a huge sigh of relief. It was all over! I hadn't really thought about the baby up until that point very much as I was just so focussed on the pain. It's like I had almost forgotten that the pain would result in this tiny little baby and because she came out from behind me I couldn't see her, so for a moment I forgot, but suddenly realised; "Wow, I have a baby." I couldn't turn myself around and over the umbilical cord fast enough to have a look at her. When I did, the midwife put a little baby in my lap and I was just overwhelmed with love and emotion, pride and an amazing sense of achievement. It must have been about 30 seconds when I realised we didn't know the sex. I was just too amazed to even ask what the sex was. I figured they would just tell me. However, they let Matt and I find out on our own. She was a girl. That was the absolute best part of all. I was crying my eyes out, so was Matt, we just couldn't believe it. A beautiful baby girl. I not only had a release from that pain, but a brand new little baby girl. It was just the best feeling in the world.

I stayed in the spa crying and crying until they asked me to get out. I didn't tear or anything, so hopping out of the spa was not painful, although I was pretty wobbly. To get the placenta out they wanted to give me an injection but I said; "No." I hate needles. So I lay down on the bed and let it come out naturally. Everything went wonderfully, I couldn't believe we had the most beautiful baby girl in the whole world; it was worth every second of pain. She was worth everything!

23 June

I have been getting period-like cramps on and off all day today, lasting for about 30 seconds each time, they are very painful, and I feel like I need to do a big poo afterwards. What is this sensation? Are they Braxton Hicks contractions? I don't think I'm supposed to have period-like cramps. Then again I have tiny different little quirky pains here and there all the time.

I have an appointment with Mrs Z tomorrow, finally. I had previously cancelled my last two appointments and it's now been five weeks since my last visit, so it will be great to see her and have a chat.

Chapter 7

Thumb up your bum...

"Somewhere on this globe, every ten seconds, there is a woman giving birth to a child. She must be found and stopped."

Sam Levenson

WEEK 30

24 June

Reading 'Prenatal Parenting' today, one line really hit me smack bang in the face. "When your unborn baby kicks, he is aggravated or anxious."

What? Aggravated? Anxious? Holy shit. My baby kicks constantly, or at least it feels like he kicks, unless he's head butting the side of my womb, which I'm sure couldn't be any better. I thought babies were supposed to kick? Upset and concerned I called Adele and asked her if babies were supposed to kick, if it was normal? To which she replied; "Did a man write that book?"

25 June

My youngest sister Peta arrived today. She is a gypsy travelling the world and has just come back from New York. Ooooohhh. It is great to have her here, as she is very excited at seeing her big sister pregnant and gives me lots of attention. She says I look a lot like Adele, which is a good sign as Adele is the same height as me and is now a tiny eight stone after she gave birth to her third child five months ago. *(It seems like I am obsessed with my weight. I AM.)*

We could not meet her at the airport to pick her up today as I had an appointment with Mrs Z. I also had another blood test. I feel like I should be a pro at this by now, dealing with pain in a civilized way *(since child birth is only 10 weeks away)* but I still had to wiggle my toes and sing funny songs to myself today until the blood test was over. I now have to go to see Mrs Z every two weeks. I hope I don't need a blood test every time, that's just ridiculous… Anyway, she checked my weight (10 stone, which means I've put on about 33 pounds now) and then I had a talk to her about the heartburn I was getting, for which she gave me a prescription. I also asked her about the dangers of the ultrasound on the baby, since we have spoken to a few people lately who think it may not be very safe. However, she reassured me that it was safe and not too worry. I then had an internal and we waited about ten minutes before she showed us our little man on the screen again. He looked so beautiful, and he kept opening his mouth. I think he was singing!

26 June

Felt quite grumpy today, plus extremely tired. It's been so hot here lately and I am sweating my tits off. To make matters worse, I decided to put some fake tan on today. Ha! What a joke. Seriously, what was I thinking? I couldn't tell half the time if I was rubbing in fake tan, or just rubbing in my own sweat.

27 June

I look like a fat leopard. My fake tan did not work, and I have very blotchy skin. I am so embarrassed, I look completely ridiculous.

I also measured myself today. Holy shit!

Waist - 39.5 inches

Hips - 39.5 inches

Bust - 40.5 inches

Thigh – 22 inches

28 June

OK. This is it! This is the feeling pregnant women go on and on about. Yes, I'm completely knackered. I hardly have any energy lately, it's fading fast and I must accept this fact instead of trying to fight it. I was supposed to call my Daddy for his birthday today, but I was just too tired. I love my Dad, but even everyday errands are becoming difficult. I had to have a nap today. I could not keep my eyes open, and I swear my body is saying; "Kelly, please… Stop… Let me rest." I can feel it, and I must pay attention otherwise I am going to be miserable. I must just accept the fact that my body really can't do what it has always done.

It's now official. I am a hippo…

I am also getting a little nervous as I am on the home stretch now and I feel I have so many things to prepare. For instance: my perineum. I have not been doing anything to stretch it. I mean how are you really supposed to stretch that tiny piece of skin between your foo and your butt hole?

A friend told me that I should stick my index finger up my minnie and my thumb up my bum, then massage the skin in between gently with olive oil. She said she did it and didn't tear at all.

Neither have I been doing those pelvic floor exercises. I always forget and anyway they are just sooooo fucking boring.

Adele told me that I should paint a small red dot on a piece of paper, cut it out, and pin it up on a wall somewhere in the house, and whenever I see it I should do my pelvic floor exercises. Good idea.

I really must start pulling and squeezing those muscles together every day if I want to have a tight vag after the birth. My husband is young and there are 20 year old girls to compete with out there. God, who said pregnancy was a piece of cake? Or was it that you are supposed to eat cake? I can't remember?

30 June

JC is on holidays for a week, very exciting, so I get to have him all to myself. We were actually hoping that he could take a bit longer off so that we could go to some tropical island and had a holiday. However, there were just too many reasons why that is not going to happen: Peta is still here, for one. I also think it's too late for this fat mamma to go anywhere. We were in London a few weeks ago, and flying at this stage of pregnancy is a bit scary. I hear so many stories lately about mothers giving birth prematurely, even as early as 25 weeks, so it seems a bit risky. I think the airlines also won't let you fly from about 34 weeks, in case you go into early labour. Shit!

WEEK 31

1 July

Went to Mrs Z for a check up today and farted in the chair just before she walked in. So embarrassed…

2 July

Yesterday Peta and I made up a dance. HA, I felt as if I was 16 again. We laughed and laughed and laughed. It was so great to let out some steam. Our dance was to a song from the Dirty Dancing soundtrack. It only lasted a minute as I was completely knackered. It was definitely a workout, and so much fun. We were supposed to video our performance, but were too busy laughing. We will have to do it before Peta leaves for London on Monday.

3 July

I can't believe how emotional I am right now. Maybe it's because the finale is drawing near, the big bang, the BIRTH! I think I am more scared than I thought I was. Because today I have cried about four times. I don't know where it all comes from? But it's so intense.

Tomorrow we are going to stay with Sue and Michael again. It's very relaxing at their house so I can't wait.

5 July

Sleeping in someone else's bed when you're pregnant is extremely frustrating. I got to sleep last night at about 6am. I could not get comfortable, and I was soooo tired. I am slightly peeved, I must admit. Aaaaargh… I really really wanted to sleep but I just couldn't. The 'itchy legs' has now spread to my hands and wrists. At one point during the night I had both my arms and legs in the air to help the circulation. *(I looked like a dead marsupial.)*

I slept in until 1pm, got up and decided before I ate anything that I would hop on Sue's scales, as the only time I can weigh myself is when I see Mrs Z, where I am weighed with my shoes and clothes on. This is not fair. Anyway, I weighed 10.8 stone this morning. So altogether I've put on 35.2 pounds since I became pregnant. *(I should have done a big poo before I even contemplated stepping on those scales.)* 35 pounds… that's 16 kegs, I mean 16 kilograms. *(I probably look like I hold the volume of sixteen kegs.)* A large bag of potatoes weighs 11 pounds each. Adele said that with her largest baby she put on 26 pounds and she is taller than me by 2 centimetres. I don't understand what I am doing wrong.

I realise that I'm having a baby, and JC constantly reminds me of this fact *(as well as telling me how beautiful I am.)* God bless him.

I know I am creating a miracle, but damn! Why can't I be one of those beautifully slender women carrying teeny tiny bumps around? Do they possess a pregnancy secret of which I am unaware?

6 July

We had a fabulous time at Sue and Michael's. However, now I have haemorrhoids, so I am happy to go home and sleep in my own big bed with my own big bum lumps.

WEEK 32

8 July

Wow, I had the most wonderful sleep last night, although I did have itchy legs again (which I will have to re-name itchy feet and ankles because it's only my feet and ankles that have that terrible feeling now.) I hate it. I know it's not painful but it's fucking annoying. Anyway, I crawled into bed around 2am, as JC and I stayed up to watch 'An American Werewolf in London' last night. Then woke up at 2:30pm in exactly the same position. How fantastic! I then got up and did a wee that lasted about six and a half minutes. It was a gorgeous sleep, and a luxury I will not have the pleasure of in around nine weeks time. Then I had some sex. I wonder if good sex counts as exercise? Because I will gladly partake of more sex if it's going to keep me fit for labour.

9 July

Went for another check up today. Had my blood pressure taken, my finger pricked *(ouch)* got weighed, and was then taken to a little room where my belly was strapped up by two thick elastic belts. Underneath each belt was what looked to me like an ice hockey puck. Then I was told to sit down and relax while the baby's heartbeat was being recorded; so sit down I did, on the most comfortable chair I've ever encountered in my adult life. Oh my God! These gynaecologists really know what they're on about. I could have stayed in that chair all day! Afterwards, I was given an internal, and JC met me in there so we could see our little man again; he is so beautiful. Though Mrs Z did say today; "Oh yes he looks extremely handsome, and look at his nose, it's very big!" Very big? Is that supposed to be a compliment in Germany? A big nose? Instantly I thought of Gerard Depardieu. I looked straight at JC. *(He has Italian blood and a big nose would come from his side of the family.)*

Mrs Z then told us that it wasn't so much long as it was wide… "Great," I thought. "So it's not Gerard Depardieu, it's more like Marlon Brando."

10 July

I am weeing about 67 times a day. Seriously, I feel like I am on the toilet every five minutes. My bladder is out of control, and I've also been feeling frightfully lazy lately. I don't want to walk anywhere; it's completely over-rated. I mean I'd like to be able to do more of it, but my feet are always attached. That's the problem.

12 July

Can someone please remind me next time I'm pregnant that I should not wear g-strings when I have haemorrhoids? They keep cutting into my asshole.

13 July

I am a beast!

WEEK 33

14 July

Today, while browsing at my personal pregnancy calendar on the net, I read some information about doing kegal (pelvic floor) exercises. "To do a kegal, tighten the muscles around the vagina and anus and hold for eight to ten seconds about 200 times a day." 200 TIMES A DAY??? If I multiply ten seconds by 200, then divide that by 60, that is 33 minutes worth of pelvic floor workout a day. Do these people realise how boring pelvic floor work is? I mean, I know it's for the good of our fannies, so we don't wee our pants before and after birth, but I guarantee that even if I **did** wet my pants one particular day, it would not take me 33 minutes to clean up the damn mess!

16 July

I have started drinking raspberry leaf tea. A lot of books recommend it, as it prepares the uterus for birth, and blah, blah, blah, so this is a good thing I guess. *(Anything that makes it easier.)* Straight up it's pretty awful, but I have been adding fresh mint, lemon and honey to it and it's actually quite nice.

18 July

I have been completely consumed by this pregnancy lately, hardly talking about anything else, and I feel as though JC is over it because I'm sure I just keep reading the same old shit to him over and over again to him.

However today I actually found something (from 'Natural remedies for morning sickness and other pregnancy problems' by Denise Tiran) which I knew would grab his attention. "If thrush develops (in pregnancy) a single clove of garlic, unpeeled to avoid stinging to the walls of the vagina, well oiled and wrapped in muslin, can be inserted into the vagina and left for two to three hours."

And grab his attention it certainly did. He said he's not going to eat garlic again, just in case I've put it up my foo.

19 July

My nails look absolutely brilliant lately. They are hard and shiny (they look a bit like my husband's bollocks without the hair.) *I am so funny...*

I've never had good nails. They've always been really soft and brittle, however, now I am actually getting long fingernails. I feel very glamorous. My hair is also fabulous. It's always shiny and I rarely have to do anything to it to make it look good. I am blessed. I guess there should be some fabulous things to counteract the bulging tummy, tits, thighs, ass, face, and batwings!!!

20 July

It is so hot, I can't believe it. I feel like I am back in Australia, except in Australia there is air conditioning.

I slept on and off for only about four hours last night. It was exhausting, I really have not been enjoying my sleep too much these last few nights.

21 July

I found out from my 'Baby Prima' magazine that the baby is now about 15.8 inches long - the exact length of my teddy bear 'Caramel', whom JC bought for me as a present last year. So today I spent about two hours dressing the teddy, putting diapers on the teddy *(actually JC did this first)*, putting teddy to bed and nursing teddy in my arms. It is so weird to think that our baby is the same size as Caramel. It is a perfect comparison, although Caramel is a bit hairier than we would like our son to be *(and Caramel doesn't look like Marlon Brando)*.

WEEK 34

22 July

My feet are as big as two bouncy castles, they are so swollen. I am amazed that they can just stay swollen all day like that. And they hurt even more than before. At night time I feel like I need to hang upside down like a vampire to sleep, just so the blood will rush to my head *(although I guess swollen feet would be better than a swollen head.)* I am also constantly complaining. I hate it, that's just not like me. I hear myself moan, and I want to hit myself, but these little aches and pains never end, not even for a minute, not when I sleep, or make love, or even take a bath. I can't escape.

I've made a secret promise to myself today to be more optimistic, to not complain as much and to concentrate on the positive aspects of pregnancy, which are, um….. Well… That the baby will be delivered by a stork at the end of this fiasco?

23 July

Today JC and I decided to go to our hospital to ask a few questions which we forgot to ask last time. We were both rather excited about visiting the hospital again and speaking to our midwife Marie. However, our excitement turned to disappointment when upon arrival a German speaking midwife told us that she was 'sorry, there was no one in the labour ward who could speak English at this time.' No Marie. No English. Nothing! This nurse was not very helpful at all and I think she thought we were actually quite rude, imposing on her time. Bitch!

Luckily for us there was an English-speaking mother lying on a trolley bed and she managed to translate for us. We told her that we had some last minute questions about the hospital, procedures and information on any new drugs that would be used in the labour. *(She did not find the last question very amusing.)* The nurse then booked us in for an appointment with an English-speaking midwife on Friday morning.

"What if you were really in labour?" JC said as we left. "There would have been no one here to communicate with us today, and that sucks." This was a valid point. It did indeed suck. What if I was in labour early and we got to the hospital and there was no one to talk to us? We are now both a bit concerned, and one of our first questions on Friday will be; "Is there an English speaking midwife available to help us during the labour and birth at any time of the day, twenty four-seven?" If not, we will need to organise a midwife to help us privately. Shit. It seems all so last minute now. However, what can we do? We were told months ago that this would not be a problem.

I am not happy.

24 July

Yesterday I bought… Ready? It's so exciting…. A brand new nightdress and three pairs of super huge undies. They are all made of cotton and soooo comfortable. I also bought some peppermint foot spray from 'The Body Shop', which is quite good, and some mandarin-flavoured lip balm to use in labour. When I got home I put my new undies on for JC and he pissed himself laughing, I started laughing too, and then it happened, I actually did piss myself…

25 July

Today we went to the hospital. It was very exciting, apart from the fact that JC and I were incredibly tired, since it was only 10am…N.B. Adele says a sleep-in for her is 8:30am, so I think we might have to start practising getting up a little bit earlier soon. Anyway, everyone at the hospital was extremely helpful today, even Nasty Midwife from a few days before. We also mentioned today that we performed in 'Starlight Express', which made us instant celebrities, so this helped. The first woman we spoke to was a midwife named Imberg *(which sounds like a type of lettuce to me).* However she was just so lovely and I've decided that I want her! Unfortunately I don't think it's up to me, but fate, and the person who writes the rotas at the hospital. She was really helpful though and answered most of our questions, our first one being;

"Will there be someone who can speak English to us when we come in for the birth?"

"There will always be someone in the hospital who can speak English here, that is not a problem." *(Yippee)*

"When I'm in labour, should we call first or just come in?"

"Just come in."

"How do you say 'contractions' in German?"

"WEHIN." *(It's pronounced Veehin.)*

"Would it be helpful if JC timed my contractions?"

"Yes please."

"Are you allowed aromatherapy oils in the hospital?"

"Yes."

"How do you say epidural in German?"

"PDA."

"Can JC stay with me all day in the hospital once the baby had been born?"

"Yes, but he will be kicked out around 10pm."

"How do you say in German; 'My vagina is tearing in two, and I am in so much fucking pain, can I go home now?'

"Sorry?" *(Forget it)*

"Do you have a fridge we could use in the midwifery unit?"

"You mean a cool box? No."

"How long for a normal labour will I stay?"

"About three or four days." *(Fabulous, sleep!)*

Imberg then finished monitoring the baby's heartbeat, I gave her a wee wee sample, and we were asked to wait for the doctor as she would answer any other questions we had.

The doctor *(very pretty with blonde hair)* was extremely nice, and spoke great English, this made both of us feel so much more comfortable and confident. I asked her;

"Can JC stay with me if I need to have a caesarean?"

"Yes, unless you have been completely knocked out by general anaesthetic, because it really won't difference since you won't know whether he is there or not at the time."

"Do you give an injection to stimulate delivery of the placenta?"

"No, we usually let it come out by itself or we administer acupuncture to certain points in your abdomen." *(This sounds groovy).*

"Do you have epidurals?"

"Yes, known as PDA."

"Do you have gas and air?"

"No, but I have heard of this in England." *(Great!)* She paused… **"Alternatively we have fantastic homeopathic tablets that help significantly with contractions and labour, and we have had much success with this."** *(Cool. Natural remedies are better, as long as they work.)*

"Do you routinely do episiotomies?"

"Only if they are necessary. It depends how flexible your perineum is, and how the baby is doing?"

"Will you give an injection for an episiotomy?"

"Not all the time, that also depends. Sometimes we have to do a cut there very quickly and we have no time to give an injection, however, your vagina is usually so far stretched at that point that the nerves surrounding your opening will be blocked from pain anyway, so you won't even feel the cut." *(Did I have to ask that question?)*

"Do you have epidurals in this hospital?"

"YES." *(Okay, now I'm satisfied).*

She then did a quick ultrasound, and we had a sneaky peak at our beautiful boy once again. She said that everything looked normal - he was growing steadily and weighs 2.5 kilogram. She then did an internal to check that my cervix was still there, and then said we were all done, and she will see us again soon.

As we casually wander back through winding corridors toward the elevators, we get the chance to take a look inside a few of the maternity rooms. There are a few women lying on their beds with large bellies hanging out, and I can't quite distinguish whether they have had their babies yet or not. But it still looks so exciting all the same. We hear babies crying in the distance and see a couple holding their new born baby in a car chair ready to take home, he is so tiny and incredibly gorgeous. All of a sudden I feel extremely jealous. I want to see our baby. I want to know what he looks like and how beautiful he's going to be. I can't wait.

26 July

I had the time to write my friend Sarah *(who is also expecting)* an email today.

Hi Sarah,

Pregnancy, what a blast! Well, I must admit, the first 28 weeks or so were just absolutely fantastic (minus the first 12 weeks of morning sickness). However we were warned of this and armed, so it wasn't too bad. Now however I am getting slightly over it. I've read all the books. I know everything there is to know about pregnancy and childbirth and episiotomies *(I even know how to spell the big words.)* So it's not so new and exciting now; it's just a bloody pain in the arse! Yes, I am venting. It's just so damn hot here which does not help things; every part of my body is rubbing together, my boobs onto my tummy, my underarm onto my boobs, the bottom of my belly onto my fanny, and my thighs onto, well, actually my legs rub together all the way from the top to the bottom. Wearing a skirt is just asking for a rash. And I've not waxed in months. For starters, I can't fucking see it, can I? And secondly, who else would be game enough to take a look down there? It's a jungle. I swear, my pubic hair is growing at a rate to rival the speed of light.

Everyday seems to last for about 56 hours, and while I am enjoying the time off, I must admit that I would be so happy if the watermelon arrived in four weeks instead of six. Soon, I will pack my hospital bag ready for the big day, and we have more or less got everything together now for the little tiger, which has been really fun. I am also having my baby shower on Monday, so that will be great. Apparently the girls have done a collection from everybody in the theatre and said I am going to score big time. Yipeee.

My belly measures 41.5 inches now, as I have been keeping measurements of all my body parts since I first got pregnant. *(I've had a lot of time on my hands to do things like that.)* My belly started off being 26.5 inches and is now 40 inches. My thighs have gone from 20.5 to 22.5 inches and my bust 34 to a whopping 41 inches. And YES I do have stretch marks. My tits look like two static globes! Luckily my stomach has no stretch marks, and I have been rubbing all kinds of creamy substances into my belly to keep it that way. I really did not want to be left with stretch marks after the liposuction I had a few years back. *(Yeah, right, like THAT was worth the effort!)*

Anyway, I should go, I hope you are really great, and everyone is looking after you well.

JC and I are both getting really excited. We know everything is going to be fabulous, and we are looking forward to meeting our new baby boy, he is going to be so beautiful. *(Although we have been told he looks like Marlon Brando from the Godfather).* Nevertheless we will love him unconditionally, as we already do.

Don't you just love your baby moving inside you? I am so random.

Please email me again soon; it is so great to hear from you.

And do you know if you're having a boy or girl? What names have you got picked out? Are you afraid of giving birth? Do you feel wonderful being pregnant? Are you over my questions?

Look after yourself Sarah, and give your baby lots of foetal love breaks...

All my love,

Kel xxx

27 July

I decided to call my girlfriend Roxanne in Australia today. It was so great to speak to her, and we chatted and laughed for over four hours on the phone. It was wonderful. I guess I won't be able to have many talks like that soon with a baby to look after? Poo. My whole life is changing. I am really going to make sure that I enjoy these last few weeks, as I know I will never have this kind of time to myself ever again. *(Wow, that really just sunk in.)*

I keep wanting this pregnancy to be over, but in reality this is the last free time I have for myself for a long time. This is the final phase of my freedom how I know it. Never again will I be able to think only of myself - my needs, my feelings, and my wants. In just over five weeks we will have a baby, who will become a toddler, then a pre-schooler, then a high school student, then someone's husband? Then a father of his

own who will one day put his mother into an old age home....
My God, I'm exhausted just thinking about it.

I wrote out my pregnancy mission statement today.
Just like Dr Whatshisface *(who wrote 'Prenatal Parenting')*
told me to.

He said; "A pregnancy mission statement should
contain all that is uniquely you, what you want during your
pregnancy, the birthing experience, and the rest of your life
with your child."

I am probably leaving it a bit late, but better late than
never, right?

Pregnancy Mission Statement

**I, Kelly O'Brien, wish to be focussed and motivated,
optimistic and enthusiastic for the remainder of this
pregnancy. It is important for me to enjoy these last few
weeks for myself, my husband and our baby by remaining
positive and happy. I want to meditate at least five times a
week to relax my mind, my body and my child, preparing
me for not only the birth but for the rest of our lives. I
want to massage my perineum every day and also practise
my pelvic floor exercises to ensure an easier and more
relaxed birth *(if that exists)*. I want to make all my own
Birth Announcement cards. *(Then again depending on
time, I may just order them over the internet.)* I want
to finish the letter I am writing to my husband telling
him how incredible he's been for the duration of this
pregnancy and how much I love him. I want to swim**

twice a week leading up to the birth and stay as physically fit as I can.

I want my birthing experience to be positive and uplifting. I wish to be in control of my own pain and use my breathing and relaxation techniques to help me with any discomfort. I wish for a happy and healthy baby. I want my body and mind to transcend all physical limitations and erupt in a mystical awakening. *(Does that even make sense?)* I want to feel at one with my partner. I want to give birth in water and feel as relaxed and focussed as possible. I want my perineum to stay in tact and my arse not to fall out. I want to feel listened to and supported by the midwives and the hospital staff. I wish the pain to be bearable, and if I need drugs I want the staff to say; 'When and how much?" I wish to hold the baby after he's born and feel overwhelming love and a special bond. I want all three of us to be surrounded by an invisible shield which protects us and gives us an amazing feeling of connection and love.

I want the rest of my life with my child to be full of happiness and laughter, joy and magic. I want us to be very close as a family and the love between JC and I to be unbreakable, as the love we share will show our son the world through our eyes. I wish our baby to grow up being loving, confident, strong, motivated, excited about life, caring, giving, beautiful and happy. He is going to be... Actually, he already is.

28 July

Last night I felt a very strange sensation. As I was bending over JC, who was lying on the couch, giving him a kiss. I stood up and felt a really heavy feeling in between my hips, which made me stand with my legs apart and take hold of the wall. I felt a shift. All of a sudden the pressure on my bladder became extremely intense, my butt felt much larger than usual and I could breathe! I mean really breathe like I used to be able to. The pressure on my heart and lungs and diaphragm was gone. Immediately I thought; "The baby's engaged." I was so excited. I then looked into the mirror and my bump had definitely moved. It was much lower. I thought; "Does early engagement mean early labour?" I popped on to the internet to find out. "No, it doesn't." For a second there I thought that maybe our baby was only a couple of weeks off, which excited me terribly. Even more exciting were the Braxton Hicks Contractions that immediately became much stronger and intense straight afterwards. They really hurt, and I was loving it…

We went to bed, and can I tell you how wonderful my sleep was? It was perfect. I was taking big deep breaths, filling my lungs with air and exhaling like a Yoga teacher. Thanks tiger!

WEEK 35

29 July

I had a baby shower tonight and it was wonderful. Danni had asked me if there was anything that we needed for the baby, and I had given her a list, but hadn't expected to get everything on that list. We got a sterilizer, a fabulous nappy bin *(which I'm told is THE best nappy bin any parents could ever wish for),* a play gym, a baby bath, some stretch suits, dummies, plastic bibs, a thermometer, baby wipes and a snug like a bug in a rug sleeping bag with arm holes, which is fantastic as babe cannot wriggle down underneath the covers.

We ate spaghetti bolognese, garlic bread and potato salad. I wish I could have eaten more but I just cannot shovel the food in like I used to. I felt ashamed being over 70kg and not being able to out-eat the other girls. I wish JC was there to share it with me, but I guess baby showers are traditional for women, and men have something else later. I will have to ask JC what that is called again *(something to do with wetting someone's head?)*

It was a wonderful evening though, and we even played a baby quiz, which was a big hit. The question which provoked the best answers was; "What is an episiotomy?"

"A piss test."

"Where it comes out your wee hole."

"Checking via your minge that everything is OK?"

And my absolute favourite; "Stitching up of the bladder."

At the end of the night a couple of the girls shared their birth stories with us all. My friend Kristy told me that the worst part of labour for her was the dry shave they gave her before they cut her perineum - details I probably didn't need to hear.

DANNI'S BIRTH STORY GOES LIKE THIS

My husband Matthew and I were living in Germany at the time, so I was quite apprehensive about the whole birth experience. It started out quite easily, however.

I was lying on the sofa talking with my mum when my waters suddenly broke. I was five days overdue and completely shocked because there was just so much water - like a water balloon had popped, and I was absolutely soaking wet.

I called my husband's work, and asked them to tell Matthew I was going into labour but not to make a big fuss as I was not experiencing any labour pains. However, a fuss was inevitable and as soon as the news broke out, everyone at Matthew's work started clapping and cheering. Then he raced off in a panic to meet me at the hospital.

Meanwhile, mum and I were getting things together. As I walked around the flat, my waters were flooding everything. The amniotic fluid was everywhere. I really couldn't believe how much water there was. We left as quickly as possible, but not before I had time to put on a face full of make up. I guess I wanted to look pretty while I was giving birth; like anyone's going to be looking at my face!

We got into a taxi and went to the hospital and when we arrived Matthew was already there waiting. We went straight to the maternity ward where the staff lead me to a room and put me straight onto a CTG machine to monitor the baby's heartbeat. After about an hour, they then took me to another little room so I could wait patiently for my contractions to really begin. (Fun.)

After half an hour or so the contractions began, and within a short space of time they started getting more and more intense. I felt like I needed to move around, so I just paced back and forth. Matthew and my Mum just sat there, which actually really annoyed me at the time. I felt like swearing at them because they weren't doing anything, and I know they were being really kind and sympathetic, but that just annoyed me even more!

After a while I was moved into another room. Then the pain started getting really strong, and they asked me whether or not I would like an epidural. To which I replied; "Absolutely, yes, now, give it me." I had to go down to the birthing room for this, but by this stage I couldn't even walk, so they wheeled me down in a wheelchair and I felt like a pregnant granny.

The next part becomes a bit of a blur because I was just experiencing so much pain. I do remember grabbing Matthew and asking him how long it would be until the epidural could be administered. In this time I had dilated very quickly to ten centimetres.

The next thing I knew they were all asking me to push. So I did, as hard as I could. I just kept pushing every time they told me to, in every damn position they could think of, including squatting on the floor (where all that happened was that I peed myself).

The midwives just kept telling me to push every time I had a contraction but I just felt pain the whole time, at the same intensity, so I really didn't know when to push at all.

After about an hour and a half the doctor came in to see what was happening because the baby obviously did not want to come out! She put her hand up my moo and tried to push my cervix back behind the baby's head but it was just too tight. They decided then that the baby would never come out naturally and I would have to have a caesarean.

At that stage I actually felt quite relieved, as I was in so much pain and felt so frustrated at having been pushing and grunting for so long. I was glad that the pain would be over soon. They also told me later that the baby's heart rate was dropping and they had to get him out as fast as possible.

So I was put to sleep and the C-Section was done. Unfortunately Matthew could not be in the delivery room, but they let him in directly afterwards to hold our beautiful son.

I woke up about two and a half hours later and they laid our baby straight on my chest which felt amazing. A tiny little beautiful baby boy.

We called our son Jacob.

30 July

I bought two maternity bras today. They're not the cheapest damn things around are they? However, they are so comfortable and undo at the front while your boob is still supported. Obviously a woman's design!

I read that you should start packing your hospital bag at week 36 (which is in six days) so I have been rushing around getting last minute items today; not fun when your swollen feet look like........

N.B. I just asked JC what was BIG and SQUISHY with which to compare my feet. He answered; "YOUR ASS." Thanks a lot!

So now I will finish the sentence...

Not fun when your feet look like your ass!

31 July

'Toe lifting' should be an Olympic sport. I would definitely win Gold. I have it perfected. I don't need to squat down anymore to pick clothes or towels off the floor, I only need to place the item in between my two biggest toes, clench together and lift. I have it down and I seem to just get better and better; today I even picked up a glass off the floor.

Went for a swim tonight and felt gorgeous in the pool, although I don't seem to be swimming as much as I am just floating. The pressure taken off my tummy, my back and my FEET is wonderful. Although I was wondering today - if my waters broke while I was in the swimming pool, would I even realise?

1 August

OK. I need to let my fears out...

I have been bottling them in and I need to release them.

Deep down I am scared that our baby will have some kind of problem. It's as if I don't think we deserve a happy, healthy baby. Everything in our lives always turns out right and great, but maybe, just maybe our baby will die or he will have special needs or a problem with his heart? I did smoke weed, I did do a few lines, and I drank too. I'm scared. I want our baby to be healthy, and I really don't like having these thoughts in case they come true. However, I must face my fears and write them down. I must get past them.

I keep reminding myself that the baby is formed now, and I'm sure he is perfect. Deep down I know he's OK. I am just living out a painful fear *(so think good thoughts Kelly, your negativity is passing through the placenta as you write this.)*

God, I really hate that fucking prenatal parenting doctor!

2 August

Last night I thought that I was going into early labour. About 15 minutes after JC and I had sex, I started getting really strong, painful contractions. Apparently there is something in semen that helps ripen the cervix? They were Braxton Hicks I know, but damn they hurt. It was about 2:30am. JC was asleep next to me and I just lay there feeling my tummy tighten and hurt every 20 minutes or so for at least an hour and a half. Secretly I was a little excited though I thought; "Maybe this is it?" So I waited for the contractions to get stronger, but they didn't and I fell asleep.

3 August

My depressing new measurements are as follows:

Waist - 41.7 inches

Hips - 40.5 inches

Bust - 40.9 inches

Thigh - 22.8 inches

4 August

That's it; I want the baby to come right now! I know he would be premature, but I'm 36 weeks tomorrow and I'm certain he would be fine. After having my intense Braxton Hicks contractions yesterday, I finally decided it was time to pack my hospital bag. It has been fun collecting the items needed for the hospital, and I have accumulated necessities based on about seven different pregnancy and birth books, so I think that I have it all pretty much covered.

My list is as follows: a dressing gown, two nighties *(one for giving birth in that I can throw away afterwards, and a pretty one for showing visitors how gorgeous I will look after the birth),* slippers and socks because apparently women in labour can get really cold feet, a towel, a hot water bottle for aches and pains, aromatherapy oils, body butter from the body shop so JC can massage me, water spray and a flannel to wipe and cool my face, lip balm, maternity Pads *(I just bought normal super pads),* two maternity bras, breast pads, big undies, nipple cream, portable CD player with CD selection, video camera which needs to be charged, normal camera, film, diary to write in *(if I can be arsed at the time),* going home clothes *(which is hard as I have absolutely no idea what I'm going to look like when I leave - I guess I will just wear maternity clothes home again, that way if I am at all a little slimmer, I will feel fantastic that my clothes are a bit baggy),* a car seat for the new member of the family, coins for long distance calls to Australia and England as we can't use mobiles *(although JC could probably just stand out the front of the hospital)* and, of course, things for baby! Plus a few items Adele told me she couldn't have done without, like a tea towel for biting into when she was bearing down *(I think that's a visual I could have done without)* and energy bars if I need a boost.

Am I scared? Yes, I am. I am scared, and excited! Reality hits so hard at times, and I actually repeat to myself; "I'm having a baby, there is a real baby inside my tummy." At times it feels so surreal, other times so mundane. I want to meet this baby that takes up so much of my space. I want to see that he's real and not just a pigment of my imagination *(yes Adele, I know it's supposed to be 'figment').* No matter how hard I try to picture him, I just can't. It's only when he moves that he seems real. However, he doesn't move quite so much anymore. I guess he has run out of space in there, and it's getting pretty tight.

Aaaahhhh. I'm sick of waiting now, and there are no new facts to read about the baby anymore. He's still getting fatter and fatter, putting on more weight every day. And if our baby did happen to come now, my foo would most definitely stay intact because he would be so small.

I have 4 weeks to go, and maybe even longer. Oh my life! How could I cope with another six weeks? This weather is unbearable. It is still so hot, and for the last two days I have just sat in the house in front of the fan with my face so close to it when I sing I sound like Britney Spears. *(I am deadly serious about this - you must try it!)*

Chapter 8

How do you spell Haemorrhoids?

"Life is tough enough without having someone kick you from the inside."

Rita Rudner

WEEK 36

26 August

I can't believe the heat...I know I keep going on about it, but it's so damn hot. A European heat wave, they call it. Today London was the hottest it's been in many years - 35.4 degrees.

7 August

Another visit to see Mrs Z today. Had to get up at about 9am, which was quite confronting. I was so tired, haven't been sleeping very well. I need to take this bloody bump off and have a good night's sleep. God, I would love that.

I am getting really excited about the birth now. I am daydreaming about how wonderful it's all going to be. I have been meditating a lot and picturing my perfect birth. I know it's all going to be great. I think also that I have quite a high pain threshold… So I'm going to give birth like 'Xena Warrior Princess', although I may take the sword out of my hand.

8 August

41 degrees today. Holy shit.

9 August

A Poem

I hate being fat when I'm pregnant, I feel like my body's not mine,

This big fucking tummy's too heavy. To be this big is a crime.

I can barely make love to my lover, and these days are hotter than hell,

I sweat like a God-damn gorilla; and feel just as smelly as well.

My face is as fat as my ass and I'm dreaming of just being slim,

I feel like I'm gonna scream and cry, or smash my husband's face in.

And if I look at another pregnant model, who's glamorous, shiny and new,

I'm gonna rip out the page, shit on her face and toss the mag in the loo.

I'm SICK of being so pregnant, I'm tired and moany and sore,

My perineum's not stretched, coz I can't be fucked doing my pelvic floor.

Who ever said it would be beautiful - to be pregnant and pretty? Oh please!

I have white blotches on my face, my tits are a disgrace, and too much fat on my knees.

I used to be gorgeous and sexy, I was a hottie, believe me it's true...

But now I have haemorrhoids bursting out my ass, and a really smelly foo.

I can't wait until I go into labour, I'm gonna push this boy out in one grunt,

Then cry when the nurses tell me that they've had to snip my "_____."

10 August

It's 4:30am. I went to bed at 12:30am and I have been up about eight times. My feet are burning up. I have put them under cold running water (although the water isn't very cold since global warming took over two weeks ago.) I've also scrubbed them with a loofah *(no good)* and tried to sleep with two cold flannels over each foot *(also no good since I keep wriggling about and they won't stay on).* At one stage I even wet two socks and wore them to bed. However, this cut the circulation off around my ankle, and made the whole thing worse. It's not fair; I want my old feet back, the ones that don't hurt, please!

11 August

I have been reading the funniest book: 'A Girlfriend's Guide to Pregnancy' by Kaz Cooke.

It is so hysterical. It's really been the best book I have read throughout my pregnancy, because it's so light hearted. It is factual as well as personal, and I just love Kaz's sense of humour. She totally rocks, and keeps me laughing non-stop.

Her book is split into 40 weeks, and every week gives a description of how big the baby is, and what's going on inside, as well as Kaz's very own commentary. To be completely honest, it was Kaz who inspired me to write this book.

Thanks Kaz - you're the best!

WEEK 37

12 August

I am sitting in front of the fan and I'm still sweating. My neck is sweaty, underneath my thighs are sweaty, my ass cheeks are sweaty and I am over it. I am over this weather and over the fact that I can't go outside and play under the tap with just a bikini on *(because I'm sure one of our nosy neighbours would just think I'm a pregnant fatagram.)*

I can hardly sleep anymore. I used to love my sleep, now I loathe it. I keep talking to the little man telling him it's quite OK for him to come early but he obviously has selective hearing. *(Must come from his dad's side.)*

13 August

Today I went and bought some aromatherapy oils for labour and birth -lavender for relaxation, clary sage to strengthen contractions and jasmine to combat anxiety and stress - all excellent for childbirth. I have spent so much money lately on bits and pieces I'm going to need for the birth, and of course for after the baby arrives. It's bloody insane how much you can spend. It's the little things put together that cost the most money. However, I feel that anything that will make labour and birth easier for me is well worth it...

14 August

It's cooled right down today, and wow I had such a fantastic sleep. Then I had to get up at 9am to go see Mrs Z again.

The waiting room at the clinic was soooo hot however, that I thought I was going to pass out! And oh my God, how long does a heavily pregnant woman need to wait? I was there for two and a half hours today. I couldn't believe it. I was so pissed off.

Firstly, as per routine I popped on the scales, not so routinely though did I tell the truth about my weight.... I lied. I was embarrassed, and I didn't want to face the reality and see how fat I really was. So as soon as I saw the digital numbers flashing past 11.5 stone I hopped off the scales abruptly. "11.3 stone," I said. I feel terrible for lying and I know that no one is going to judge me, but I didn't want to know how much I really weighed. I knew I wasn't over 11.5 stone, because it kept flashing between 11.3 up to 11.5, but I just didn't want to know… Ignorance is bliss. If the scales say I'm only 11.3 then my subconscious will make it so. Adele told me that I would stop putting on weight around now, HA! She also said that I would that I would slim right down after the birth by breastfeeding like she did *(that better not be another lie or I will sue)*.

There was a positive note to my appointment today. I was able to see our little man on a brand new space-shuttle-looking ultrasound. Mrs Z was able to show us a photo of his face in 3D. It was even skin coloured! His features were so well defined, I couldn't believe my eyes. He looked like a real baby. I am so excited. I want to meet him. He's my angel.

15 August

Oh my God! So much masturbating, so little time…

16 August

I have haemorrhoids again. I think it's the pressure of the baby pushing down on my bum hole. I hate them, they are so uncomfortable. I told Adele about it the other day, and she told me I was lucky. She had thrush the whole way through her second baby's pregnancy. To be honest, I don't know what's worse. Anyway, I decided to try the garlic up my bum tonight before I went to bed. And, um…Well I don't know what to say apart from OOOUUUUCCCHHHH…. I know I said this was meant to help, but I lied. I did exactly what the book said. I got the garlic, then took off the skin, tied some cotton around it, and up it went. But the pain.

Oh my God. It stung so much. I couldn't push it out quick enough. I am **not** trying that again!!

17 August

JC and I locked ourselves out of the house this morning, leaving not only our keys inside but our money as well, so we couldn't even catch a cab home from the theatre tonight. Aaarrgghh….

We therefore had to walk all the way home, which was like slow torture. I walked like an old nana the whole way, as JC ran ahead of me so that he would be home by the time the locksmith arrived. What I did notice today (other than the 80 year old grandfathers with pacemakers walking faster than me) was that my thighs (having worn a dress today) do not rub together anymore. I used to give myself a kind of beard rash before. Now the fat between my thighs just sticks together. My legs stay joined at the top near my punaani all the way down to my knees. I guess this is how mermaids feel. Except they're beautiful, and have dolphins as friends.

I also started feeling rather weird today. I experienced a brand new sensation. Everything just felt so different. It was like a transition from being 'overly heavily pregnant' to being 'so ripe that I just couldn't see the light anymore pregnant', and whilst walking past a German sausage stand I involuntarily burst into tears. I couldn't bare it anymore. The tiny steps, the massive bump, the overgrown thighs… No, it wasn't even about the physical aspects of pregnancy; it was just a feeling of vulnerability. Being a vessel for another life, like my own life just didn't matter anymore. I started getting the shakes, and realised that I probably needed some food, but there were no shops open… So I tried to walk home as fast as

I could, all the while sobbing and feeling so completely low I dragged my bag along the ground beside me like a sad little school girl. I had no intention of trying to make myself feel better; I wanted to feel shitty and sad, sorry and lost. I wanted to feel like a child. I wanted someone to look after me.

Then I got even sadder when I realised that soon I will be the one who is doing all the looking after. No one to look after me anymore... That time is over.

I forget sometimes that as soon as I give birth I will be forever an adult - the caregiver, the mother, the responsible parent, the real grown up.... My youth will be gone, and I will never again be a little girl.

18 August

The good news is that I am sleeping quite well. Bad news is everything else I say and do. I am changing. I am changing from Louise Hay into Mummy Dearest. I am turning mad. JC keeps laughing at me, and luckily doesn't take most of what I say to heart, thank God. Everything is annoying me! I feel like time is running out of my life, yet I'm desperate to have this baby. I go from moments of excitement to moments of fear and anxiety within seconds. I feel euphoric one minute then the next, feel as though I've popped 42 Es the night before and am coming down like a bitch...Oh, it's awful. There are so many things that I want to do but I just cannot move, or think, or talk or contemplate anything other than this bloody baby. I haven't been doing my pelvic floor and am wetting my pants everyday. I have not been massaging my perineum like I promised myself I would because lately I've been thinking about getting an epidural to diminish the pain and just have the whole birth pain and worry-free (if that kind of birth exists). I was really thinking positively about having a natural birth, but lately I am just so tired of being pregnant and sore and uncomfortable, I just want it to be over. I just want to hold our baby in my arms and have him here, as soon as possible. Fuck pregnancy. Oh and on that subject…. I can barely even do that anymore.

WEEK 38

19 August

It's my mamma's birthday today. I thought about being induced for her so I didn't have to buy her a present, but decided it was too much hassle. A homemade card and a long chat on the phone would have to suffice.

Oh, and I worked out why the garlic up my bum didn't work the other day. I was supposed to wrap the clove in muslin cloth *(whatever that is)* not put it up my tooshy fresh. No wonder it stung like hell.

20 August

Today I decided to write one of my last group emails since the baby could come any day now.

Email no. 3

Hello Friends, and how is everyone? I am hot, my belly is hot, my fanny is hot, my ass is sweating, my tits

are sagging, and my thighs have moulded together. A heatwave, they call it! Well, I tell you right now, this country needs to install some air conditioning because it's not natural what is happening in Europe. It is so hot I can hardly see what I'm writing because there is sweat dripping into my eyes (since I have to keep the fan blowing constantly on my noony). I think it's about 41 degrees today. Great for those who are enjoying the sun, but not for me who has now gained 39.6 lbs, piles, and a distinct waddle. I can hardly move.

Sadly I must inform you that this could be one of the last group emails I write for a very long time. My life is about to change drastically and I know I will never have this kind of time to myself again. I am 38 weeks, and they say my tummy could erupt any day now and I am wishful thinking that the baby will come early, as it is just too damn hot.

I am really looking forward to giving birth, just because I am so uncomfortable. Maybe I was naive at the beginning, but I thought pregnancy would be just a lot of sitting on the couch eating cream buns and ice cream while your husband massaged your feet! Well, I ate the cream buns and the ice cream (you can see the remains of this on my ass) and my husband does massage my feet sometimes, but he is usually too sore himself (having to do the show every night) to massage very often, let alone with enthusiasm.

I have loved being pregnant though, it has been a wonderful time, completely transforming, emotional and intriguing. However, I must admit, truthfully, I'm over it now. I mean it was gorgeous for the first 28 weeks or so but then Mother Nature turned into Mother Fucker and showed me her wrath.

Swollen feet and toes, pigmentation on my face, a long line running from my fanny to my breast bone. (What is that anyway? Is it so the doctors at the hospital can do lines of cocaine on your belly before they perform a C section?) Cellulite on my knees, and stretch marks on my boobs, complete with the darkest areolas one has ever seen outside of the Chaka Zulu tribe.

Little things I took for granted have become major feats: washing the dishes at the kitchen sink, as I have to turn sideways; picking things off the floor as I can't bend over, but have to squat, and feel like I'm doing a pee in the bush; trying to trim my pubic hair and almost taking off my clitoris! I can't even have sex with my husband anymore. It's becoming a major Olympic sport, and getting harder and harder to manoeuvre myself into appropriate positions. Even if I sit on top I feel like a sumo wrestler pinning down his opponent (not sexy!) Surprisingly though I am still as randy as a dog on heat (all those extra pregnancy hormones) and can thankfully keep masturbating three or four times a day. Unfortunately though, no sex! You must also remember that I haven't been drinking, smoking, even taking paracetamol for the last nine months. I'm a fucking nun. And sex was the only thing that kept me sane and fulfilled and now it is just an old memory fading off into the distance (along with my old figure and the infamous cigarette trick).

Anyway, my breasts have another job to do now, that of breast feeding. Won't that be weird?

I am feeling a little apprehensive about THE BIRTH.

I can feel the clock ticking away, and I am completely at the mercy of Mother Nature; I mean, we can be late at work, we can fail to meet a deadline, we can decide when or if to visit friends, even when to keep going when a stinking cold makes us bed ridden. But pregnancy has its own timetable and seasons, and this baby will come when it's damn good and ready, and I in turn must be ready also. It's a scary thought, but also completely exhilarating. I am determined to give my best shot at doing the whole natural thing. However, if the pain becomes too intense I'm not going to be Xena Warrior Princess, just a 'Princess' and ask for that nice numbing epidural. That's why it was invented wasn't it? However, no matter what happens, I'm sure I will be fine. I mean I've gone through two plastic surgery procedures, skate school, Spice Power and a break up with Simon Lind, I'm sure I can get through this...

Yes, we are getting very excited about the birth of our son (although we are still disagreeing on names!) JC likes Jacquin (pronounced JACK-WIN, not WA-KEEN) and I like Jude... I keep telling him there is no song called 'Hey Jacquin' but he doesn't seem to give a shit.

Anyway, I have attached some photos of my overgrown belly, and I really hope you enjoy them as much as I enjoyed every jam doughnut I consumed in that time... (N.B. There also is a baby in there, don't forget.)

I will write another email as soon as I have the time, (probably in another 18 years or so). No, seriously I will write when the baby is home and I have a bit of energy (probably in about three years or so…)

I hope everyone is fantastic, enjoying themselves, enjoying life and making the most of everyday. I send my love and laughter to you all, and please write when you have time, it is always great to hear from you.

So, wish me luck, and I will let you all know when little Jude/Jacquin arrives.

I love you all and think of you everyday.

God bless you (and my tearing vagina).

Love Kel xxx

21 August

Last night I excitedly thought I might be going into labour, and I was very happy.

JC and I had sex and 10 minutes later I started getting quite full on contractions again. I started timing them, and was getting myself extremely worked up at the prospect of being able to give birth 10 days early.

The first contractions were both 13 minutes apart, so I was almost wetting my pants with excitement, then however, they changed, eight minutes, 11 minutes, 16 minutes apart, DAMN! I can't believe how absolutely ready I felt. Far out, it's not fair; I really want to have this little tiger now. I guess he just doesn't want to come out yet. He's warm and snug, cosy and happy inside. He's not going anywhere.

Why do I feel like I'm really going to be pregnant forever? I have been having strong Braxton Hicks contractions for a few days now, on and off, and I cannot believe how excited I feel. I feel wonderfully ripe and ready; I want him to be here now, right now! Our little baby, our little baby who still has no name – which, by the way, is really starting to piss me off. Our baby doesn't have a name. I feel anxious about this. *(To be completely honest, I feel anxious about everything lately.)* I feel anxious that the house is constantly messy, when it looks the same as it always has. I feel anxious that I will never again look glamorous and thin. I feel anxious that I still can't eat runny eggs.

I just feel fucking anxious.

22 August

I defrosted the freezer today. I am obsessed with having a clean house at the moment. Nesting, I think it's called. I can feel myself going slightly loopy, and I can't keep still. Why do I have so much energy? I feel full of beans, ready for anything.

Ouch, OK. Having a Braxton right now! It's kind of a good pain though.

I am also OBSESSED about recognising the symptoms of labour, every time I have mild back ache, or two Braxton Hicks in a row, I automatically think; "This is it, this is labour." Boy am I wrong! It's just me being neurotic and excited and obsessed. It's very hard to think about anything else lately, and even though I'm not officially due for another nine days, I know that our little tiger is full term now, and could come any day.

23 August

I really need to have my bikini line waxed before the birth. I am so damn hairy and I need it to look nice. When can I do it? And more importantly WHO can do it for me? My friend Chantelle has offered to do it, but I'm not sure. Maybe I'm embarrassed that it's too hairy?

24 August

I just cleaned the entire house and it looks fantastic. I cleaned everything. At first I just started to vacuum, then I began cleaning behind things *(something we know we should do, but never do)* then I dusted the ceilings, cleaned the tiny grooves in the floorboards and the window sills and removed all the marks on the walls throughout the house - even the blinds!

Brilliant. Actually I did more than clean; I rearranged the furniture and redecorated. And it only took me two hours. I was an interior designer on speed.

25 August

Measurements:

Waist - 43.3 inches

Hips - 41.3 inches

Bust - 40.9 inches

Thighs - 23.5inches

Chapter 9

Don't give a German Midwife scissors...

"If pregnancy were a book they would cut the last two chapters."

Nora Ephron (Heartburn, 1983)

WEEK 39

26 August

I walked for over an hour today. My friend Gavin and I went to an old second hand furniture shop. It took us about twenty minutes to walk there, one hour to look around and about 40 minutes to walk back. I was so exhausted by the time I got home that I just passed out on the bed for three hours. When I woke up I'd wet my pants.

27 August

A Poem

Pelvic floor, pelvic floor, why are you so boring?
I'd rather stick a pencil in my eye.
Pelvic floor, pelvic floor, you know you are so boring!
Thinking of you only makes me cry.
I hate to squeeze my fanny lips together, and hold the walls of my vagina in.
Pelvic floor, pelvic floor, why are you so boring?
Please God, make pelvic floor a sin...

28 August

I keep wetting my pants and think my waters are breaking. I have been doing my pelvic floor about twice a week, but obviously it's not enough.

I got up at 1:30pm today. Yesterday I got up at 3pm. I feel so guilty. I feel like I should be practising getting up earlier for the baby. Then again, maybe I should just enjoy the sleep in and not analyse it all so much. I am so crazy lately, and due in three days. OMG, I am so ready. Baby, come out now! I feel as though I'm not even human anymore. I am tired and worn out. I am sick of being fat and I want to see my old body again.

BLAH!!!

Regardless of my whinging however, I have actually enjoyed this pregnancy *(especially the masturbating)*. It has been fascinating and amazing - not only for my body but for my mind as well. This transformation has been unbelievable. I mean, I thought puberty was difficult.

I am just eager to get rid of this bump and sleep on my tummy again, make love to my husband like a sexy woman, and not walk around like a duck. I am very excited about seeing our little man, and I am even excited about giving birth, I'm sure it will go amazingly *(trying to convince myself here)*. The time is almost here. Aaaaarrrrggghhhh!!!!

29 August

OK, exciting news. I am in the hospital right now, writing this with a drip in my hand *(which is somewhat uncomfortable.)*

It seems that my waters have broken and I have now been here for about eight hours. I don't feel any pain at all - OK, maybe a bit of period-like pain I guess - and I am one centimetre dilated. *(Only nine more painful centimetres to go.)* The midwives asked me earlier if I wanted to be induced tonight but JC and I have decided we would rather wait until the labour starts naturally.

The hospital staff told JC to go home and get some rest because we will both need it for the morning, so I am alone and I guess I have a long time to wait. I am feeling good though, really positive and sooooo excited. I cannot believe it, the day has finally arrived. I am going to have a little baby in my arms within the next 24 hours *(let's hope!)*

Anyway, it started like this today:

This morning I had an appointment with Mrs Z only to be told; "No the baby is not ready to come out yet, and come back on your due date on 3 September, then every two days after that…"

I was absolutely shattered; I had been feeling like the baby was getting ready to pop out any day. I was so upset. I thought; "Oh my God, I'm going to be pregnant forever, and definitely overdue." So grumpily I walked home feeling completely sorry for myself. When I got there JC was still in bed sleeping, so I went to the toilet and decided to get back into bed with him. It was about 3pm *(and yes, my husband was being a lazy bastard)*. Just as I was about to hop in however, I felt water dripping down my leg. "Shit, I've just wet myself again, look at the floor," I said. There was a puddle on the carpet, so I woke JC.

"Fuck, have your waters broken?" he asked

"I don't know?"

I then asked him to grab me a pregnancy book from the shelf so I could read what it said, as I wasn't sure whether I had peed myself or my waters had broken.

The book said;

"Amniotic fluid will smell and taste different than urine."

"OK", I said, "I'm gonna have to taste it."

So there I was on my hands and knees smelling the water on the floor, praying to God that it wasn't wee! Then I wet my finger and tasted it. It was sweet. It wasn't urine. "Holy shit", I thought. "I'm gonna have a baby."

I felt so excited, so nervous, so scared, so amazing, so petrified, so full on.

JC got our things together *(but not before he rolled himself a joint, mind you)*. I was in no pain whatsoever, but had to lie down straight away (since Mrs Z told me to lie down if my waters broke in case of infection.) Then we called a taxi, and made our way to the hospital where they told me; "YES, your waters have broken." I was in the first stage of labour. I was so excited. I thought; "This is it, this is really it." I was just completely overwhelmed.

That was four hours ago. Now it's 9pm, and I feel really incredible.

Anyhow, I am going to try and sleep now. I have told JC that I will call him the minute I feel pain, and he is going to come to the hospital straight away.

Wow, oh my God, I am so excited *(and a bit scared)*. Soon my whole life will be different *(and so will my foo foo)*. Please God, let my fanny stay intact and go easy on the whole pain thing OK?

Chapter 10

Epidurals Don't Work...

"I realize why women die in childbirth - it's preferable."

Sherry Glaser

WEEK 40

3 September

I am sitting here right now like a puffy watermelon. I feel like I've been hit by a truck. Like I'm in a dream. Next to me, as I write this, is a tiny baby laying in a cot beside me. His name is Oscar. I am a mother.

Finally I have the time to write everything down.... But where do I start?

Well, labour was...

To be honest...

A cunt!

An absolute fucker.

I don't know who I thought I was going to be? Mother Nature... Mother Theresa... Mother Earth? Because it was completely opposite to the kind of birth I thought I was going to have. Maybe I visualized it too many times for reality to actually be in the equation?

I will now try to put everything together piece by piece.

N.B. The story that is about to be told is a very painful one, so if you are imagining a birth surrounded by rainbows and bunnies, skip to the end...

KELLY'S BIRTH STORY GOES LIKE THIS

I fell asleep around 12am on that first night in hospital only to be woken up at about 3am with contractions - like small bursts of period pain. I decided to wait and call JC so he could get a bit more sleep, but by 6am I was in quite a lot of pain so I called him. "Baby, you need to come to the hospital, I need you here now." He didn't answer, and just hung up the phone *(unintentionally, I hope)*. **He had fallen back to sleep.**

I understand he really is not a morning person, but Oh my God, what complete and utter fucked timing! I couldn't believe it. He had even left the phone off the hook so I couldn't call back.

About 7:30am he had worked out what was going on and called me.

"Kel..."

"Don't bother coming, I don't want you here," I erupted down the phone.

"I am so sorry baby," he said. "I didn't mean to fall back asleep."

"I don't care," I screamed. "Fuck off." I was distraught and so upset. *(He arrived at 7:42am.)*

At 10am they decided things were moving quite slowly and they asked if they could get things started. I said yes. Firstly they gave me acupuncture in three different areas - just by my thumbs, in my knees and on the outside of my little toes, and boy, did this certainly bring on those contractions. Oh my God!!!

Firstly however, I must explain what contractions feel like, because I thought they would just feel like a bad period. However, they are much more intense than that, and so fucking painful. They squeeze your whole body really tight, and you can feel the pain everywhere, not just in your tummy, but all over. It's just so fucking horrible. Anyway, all of a sudden I thought to myself; "Oh my God, I really do not want to do this anymore..."

Then the real pain started...

I was then given two bottles of water up my bum, which felt disgusting and was followed by even worse contractions. I had to race straight to the toilet so I could shit myself and I began to cry. I remember sitting there in so much pain thinking about normal women having brunch with champagne talking about 'Gucci Gucci Goo', while I sat hunched over on the toilet like Big Foot. *(I was quite hairy since my friend was not able to wax my bikini line before I went into hospital.)* I was so upset, I felt disgusting sitting there, having severe contractions, diarrhoea, and sweating like a beast.

It was 12pm and I knew right then that I wanted to have an epidural. The midwife said I couldn't, as I was not dilated enough. Bitch! She said it might stop the labour if I did. SHIT! So instead she gave me a green homeopathic capsule to put up my bum. It stung so much, but it did settle the pain for a few hours, and JC and I were able to lie down and fall asleep together.

At 2pm I woke and the pain was getting worse. I asked for another green capsule, which this time was a bit like putting a green smartie up my ass for all the good it did. It just wasn't working... The pain was getting more extreme. I had almost forgotten that contractions are supposed to get more intense as labour progresses. I was not happy when I remembered this fact.

How much was this going to hurt?

I wanted something else for the pain; I needed something for the pain. And after an hour of walking around, having a sob and trying to control it, I asked for something else, anything to help. By this time, our favourite midwife Imgard had started her shift, and I was soooo happy to see her. However, my happiness subsided when Imgard appeared from behind her cupboard with the longest injection I've even seen in my life, similar to something they use in a dental surgery but as long as a poker stick. I shook my head and cried; "No, No, I don't want that." *(She was planning to inject it in my ass.)* At that moment, the doctor *(who looked like Michelle Pfeiffer)* arrived and told me that if I wanted the pain to lessen I should really have the injection. So holding my breath and squeezing JC's hand, I took it. However, lessen the pain it did not. Instead the pain increased, and that's where the shit really hit the fan! *(Well it would have if I had any shit left.)* Before I knew it, I was in so much pain I thought I was going to punch Michelle Pfeiffer in the face.

"You've GOT to be kidding, no one told me it would be THIS painful," I thought. I was trying to breathe, doing everything I'd read about in the books. JC sat by my side helping me count and focus on my breathing. However it was no good, nothing was working.

"I don't want to be in this much pain," I cried. "Isn't there anything else you can give me?" The pain was coming in waves, every three minutes it seemed. "Please, please give me an epidural now," I asked painfully. "I can't take much more of this."

"Yes, OK. We will call the anaesthesiologist out from his house now," Imgard replied.

"WHAT?" I snapped. "He's at home? I'm going to die before he arrives."

I couldn't believe it! The anaesthetist was NOT in the hospital. He had to drive all the way here? What if he had a car accident on the way? What if his car didn't start? I was getting frantic. I needed the pain to go away immediately. I couldn't comprehend how fast it was moving. It had a tight hold over my body squeezing it, hurting it, torturing it. I tried my best to keep breathing in and out, counting in and out, but as the pain crescendoed, my breaths were short and tight, it was so hard to control myself, and all I wanted to do was scream. JC was coaching me and saying all the right things (which were coincidentally all the wrong things) and just then he started stroking my face. "Don't touch me, please don't touch me!" I screamed.

Michelle Pfeiffer then bent down beside my ear and in a very calm, soft, almost angelic voice she whispered; "You are doing so well Kelly."

"No I'm not, I'm not, I can't handle it," I replied.

"Yes you can," she said. "You are so brave, you are really brave."

I remember at that point I felt quite amazing, and I calmed down a little and concentrated on my breath.

"How long until the epidural man gets here?" I asked JC.

"In 15 minutes babe," he replied.

"In 10 minutes babe," he would continue.

"In five minutes babe."

Then…

Finally, he arrived.

Mr Catwalk.

I call him that because he walked in as if he were on a bloody catwalk, casually taking his jacket off and waltzing in with an air of grace and prestige about him, and I remember wanting to punch his fucking face in. He was taking so long, and he obviously knew I was in a great deal of pain. What a cunt! He then asked me in a strong German accent; "How are you?"

"How AM I?" I thought. "How would you feel if someone skinned your bollocks and put them in a bowl of Dettol, you prick?"

I felt like an animal, a fat, hairy, sweating, moaning, grunting animal who was scared shitless (*but nevertheless thankful that Mr Catwalk had finally come to my rescue*).

Right then, he asked me to sit on the edge of the bed with my spine curved, hunched over as much as possible. "Now stay very still," he said firmly. "Do NOT move!"

I could hear the seriousness in his voice and all of a sudden, all I could picture was me, sitting in a wheelchair holding my baby. So I sat there, like a statue (with tears in her eyes, whimpering!)

I hardly felt a thing when he inserted the injection into my spine.... To be quite honest, the contractions were just too painful.

I thought the epidural would work straight away, but it didn't. I was still in pain. I kept asking; "How long? How long until it kicks in?" To which Mr C casually replied; "Very soon, very soon." However, soon did not come quick enough and I experienced five or six more contractions before the pain started to dull. And when it did.... Oh my God. There was hope in my heart. I could breathe. My heart rate slowed, and I could feel the pain lessen. It was amazing. The pain was really going away. I was so happy. I thought; "At last, I am going to be able to be really present here, I can probably even enjoy my baby being born." Up until this point, I had almost forgotten that there was a baby there at all. The pain had just been so intense and so real that all I was thinking about was how much I was hurting. I really did not think pain like that existed... Pain so bad that I thought at any moment I could die.

However, I was just so thankful now that the pain that was washing over my body was vanishing. I felt the pain subside first in my back, then my stomach, then my butt. It was truly remarkable. I thought my legs would go completely numb, but they didn't. And just for a second I thought to myself; "I need more, I need more epidural, it's not enough." The pain was still there, it had definitely lessened, but it was still there.

"I need more," I said quickly.

"No, no, you've had enough," Mr Catwalk answered sternly.

"But you don't understand," I persisted, "I took a lot of acid and ecstasy in my 20's, maybe my body is immune? Maybe I need more than the average person?"

"No, no," he responded. "This is enough for you."

Wanker.

He then proceeded to tell me how epidurals were not supposed to completely numb you, that was actually a 'falsehood' they are only meant to 'give relief, not conquer it.'

"Well... slap me fucking silly and call me Susan," I said. "I thought conquering was exactly what they were supposed to do."

"You will be fine," he said. "Soon your baby will be born." He then got his things, put on his jacket and cat-walked the hell out of there.

Just like that... He was gone.

Right then my heart started beating faster. My breathing sped up, and I began to cry.

I knew something was not right. And within five minutes, the pain that I thought was disappearing, was coming back, first in my stomach, then my bottom and then in my back.

I couldn't believe it! The pain, it was all returning.

I started to lose control of myself. *(So much for all the damn meditating and that stupid pregnancy mission statement.)* I started crying. "The pain is coming back, please, do something, it's not working," I protested. All of a sudden, Imgard, three other midwives and Michelle Pfeiffer all came running to my rescue. They were telling me to push whenever I felt a contraction, but the contractions were non-stop and I couldn't tell where one started and one ended, it all just felt the same. There was no break, just pure pain.

"Just keep pushing," they were telling me.

"Push Kelly, push."

I was pushing as hard as I could. I was pushing with all my might.

JC leaned over me. "Honey, your baby's going to be born soon, it will all be over soon, just keep pushing!"

"I don't give a fuck," I screamed. "And it's not OK, I'm going to die here."

I couldn't look ahead, or look forward. I was immersed in the pain, was part of it, and I couldn't comprehend making sense of what was going on or that it was for a good cause. I was consumed with agony coming in from every direction in all dimensions. I was losing control.

Just then, Michelle Pfeiffer came to my side again and seemed extremely concerned. She leaned into me softly and said; "Listen carefully Kelly, your baby is distressed. For your baby, you need to slow down and breathe with me, breathe with me OK? In... Hold and out... In and out." I was scared, and I tried my hardest to slow my breathing down because my baby was in danger. I started counting with her 'One.... Two... Three...'. I cried. It helped, the breathing really helped. I knew I had to do what she said. I knew there was no way the pain would end unless this baby came out.

But the pain was still unbearable. "Give me a Caesarean, please," I pleaded. *(Apparently this is when the staff know the baby's about to come out).* "The pain will stop soon I promise," said Michelle. "Not in hours, but in minutes, I promise, in minutes."

This gave me hope. I kept pushing.

Then there were five women around me. I had two midwives pushing against each leg, one woman staring into my minge, Michelle Pfeiffer at my ear, and another woman, who all of a sudden came up next to my tummy and put her hands on top of it and then began pushing down hard with all her might. Oh my God. I couldn't believe what she was doing to me! It hurt like hell itself. I felt like I was going to vomit. I cried harder as she pushed down on my fundus again and again. She was using all her body weight to push the baby out. I couldn't believe it? I'd never read about *this*. She was killing me.

"Stop it.... You're hurting her," JC yelled.

I was crying uncontrollably and immersed in pain, but I kept pushing and pushing, crying and screaming.

Then, all of a sudden, a lady appeared with a vacuum cleaner in her hand *(it could have been the cleaner for all I know)* and I could feel her putting her hands on either side of this huge bowling ball that lay perched inside my vag. All the while I was breathing and crying and breathing and swearing and pushing, and shaking, and...

All of a sudden...

The pain stopped.

Just like that. It was gone.

And there in Imgard's hands, was a little baby.

I couldn't comprehend it.

It was amazing...

A tiny little perfect baby.

He wasn't even crying, just shaking a bit with a cone shaped head, and so gorgeous. She put him straight on my belly and it was the most magical feeling. The pain was gone, all of it, just like that, so quickly. And now lying on my skin was a tiny baby *(that I had almost forgotten I was giving birth to) just* breathing quietly and quivering.

Unbelievable.

What a full on mind blowing trip. I had just gone from feeling the most terrifying pain in my life, to feeling the most joyous feeling in my life within seconds. God... how insane, and how incredible!

As soon as they put him on my tummy I thought; "Oscar". It was the perfect name for him. My beautiful Oscar. He looked shattered. I guess he had been through quite an ordeal himself.

And now, finally, after 40 weeks we meet.

A beautiful boy. My beautiful Oscar.

The time was 5:53pm.

JC started crying, and was just beside himself with pride. He kept kissing my forehead, and watching Oscar with amazement. It was the most beautiful moment.

"Thank you, thank you," I cried to all the staff. *(However, thinking about it….. it was the cleaner and I who really did all the hard work)*.

All the while, the midwives were fussing about down by my fanny, and I presumed they were delivering the placenta, which they did very quickly.

Michelle then handed some scissors to JC and asked him if he wanted to cut the umbilical cord.

"No thanks," he replied. I think JC was a little freaked out by it all. *(It was also pretty messy and bloody. I wouldn't have the cut the damn cord either.)*

What I soon realised however, was that they were also stitching me up!

"Oh my God, I've been cut," I said. I didn't even realise. I didn't feel a thing. Thank goodness!

I couldn't feel them stitch me up either. *(I guess that's where the epidural did work.)*

"How many stitches am I getting?" I asked.

"About 10," Ms Pfeiffer replied.

"Can I go out for a cigarette please babe?" JC asked.

Imgard then took Oscar over to the scales - 8 ounces, 8 grams.

"Good size," she said.

"And my foo foo knows it," I replied.

She dressed Oscar in some tiny blue baby clothes. The ones I had seen laid out on the cupboard when we first visited the hospital, and I started to cry.

I was so happy. I had done it. I had given birth. And I was so proud of myself *(even though I completely lost it and feel as though I will need some major therapy in a few weeks).*

I stared at Oscar. He was so beautiful, and so perfect. He was a bit wrinkly, and his head looked funny, but to us he was incredible.

I am now a mum. After ten months of pregnancy and 12 hours of labour.

It all seems so surreal. But here he is, our sweet little Oscar.

I cannot believe it. I am really a mother.

This journey has been so amazing. Everything seems to make so much sense now. Oscar makes so much sense. Having this tiny baby lying next to me puts everything into perspective. I don't care that I'm fat and flabby anymore. I don't care about becoming a star *(even though I probably will be.)*

I don't even care that my minge has been sliced or about the massive haemorrhoids I have while I sit here on a rubber ring with an ice pack on my anus.

All I care about is being a good mother. And being a mother feels so good. I also think it's cool now. It's cool to be a mum. And Oscar is so fabulous. I feel so blessed.

Thank you Oscar, you've helped me realise what is truly important!

My last poem
(Sung to the tune of "I Will survive")

When my contractions started I was petrified,
Didn't give a shit that my husband was by my side.
I spent the whole bloody night thinking; "How could this go on?"
I was not strong, 10 hours of pain is just too long...

And my poor back was out of place,
Even told JC to fuck off, cos he put a flannel on my face.
I was in so much pain, I had to cry,
I had to stumble cos when I walked thought I might die.

Oh, yes I…I did survive,

But there is no way that I will give birth again, as long as I'm alive.

Those bloody doctors cut my minge from the inside

I did survive,

I did SURVIVE!!!

Yeah, Yeaaaaah…..

10 September

Looking back on the birth I feel like I was on LSD. And as amazing as it was, I feel as though I've been in a horrific car accident. The birth was much worse than I thought it would be.

Maybe it was because I didn't go to Lamar classes, maybe it was because I thought I could transcend the pain? Maybe I was so focussed on it being the most amazing experience in my life I hadn't thought seriously about the pain enough at all.

God, how fucking awful childbirth can be…

I have since found out that while I was in labour, Oscar was in distress because he couldn't get out. My cervix was too small, and I probably should have been given a caesarean, but there was just not enough time *(because 30 hours isn't long enough)*. That's why that bitch of a midwife was pushing down so hard on my stomach; she had to get the baby out as soon as possible. The epidural was also put in the wrong place. It was either injected a little too high, or too low. Fuck. I guess I should just be happy that I can still walk really!

My tits are absolutely huge, they are so big I feel like they are about to explode with milicon *(milk and silicon).* They hurt soooo much, I can't bare it.

So much has changed.

The feelings I have for JC now are different. He has experienced the best and the worst with me. We will forever be bonded by what we experienced together in that delivery room. It was our blood being born, our son. We created him together, and I will love JC until the end of time. Love is the most powerful, magical gift. I had Oscar because I was so in love with a boy. That boy became my husband, and now he is a father. He is also my best friend. He was amazing in there, and he is so proud. The proudest father ever, and he can't stop kissing Oscar. He is as in love with our son as I am.

I also feel extremely protective, and my heart pounds every time Oscar makes a sound, he is just so tiny. So pure. I have never experienced this kind of feeling before. My heart is living outside of my body. Wow! What craziness? How incredible childbirth is. It's just such an intense, amazing transformation of yourself, and the new role you are about to play is terrifying and so exciting.

I already love my son, he is so beautiful. I cannot stop staring at him. I feel so blessed that he is ours.

He was worth every inch of pain I went through. And now, funnily enough, the pain is gone. I can still remember it, but I don't feel it now. Childbirth takes a day out of your life. Just one day.

And now a brand new journey is about to begin.

But that, my friends, is a whole new book…

Thank you

God, who would I like to thank? Well… I'd like to thank God actually. (I know this is the first person Whitney Houston always thanks, but I really do feel this is who comes first.)

God (The Universe, Love, Higher Power) - I don't ever really go to church, but I know you exist in some form or another. You always believed that I would finish this book (even if it did take me five years) and I did. Thank you.

Mum and Dad - Thank you for your continued support and love, for always pushing me to strive for my best and for never wanting me to be anything other than myself! You have always known that I would be your star. I love you both so much. You are wonderful parents and AMAZING grandparents!

Adele - Thank you for all your valuable information. You are such a wonderful mother and amazing kindred spirit, full of love and light. I love you so much. (To Matt, Jazmyn, Levi and Noah - thanks for being such a great family.)

Peta - You know you rock! I love you so so much and we will always be best friends.

Jean-Claude - Thank you for sharing this incredible experience with me. You were always supportive, and are a fantastic father. I will always love you and know that we will always be friends (and wonderful parents).

Sylvia - Thank you for your open mindedness, carefree spirit, calm nature and listening ear. You are treasured deeply. I love you. Thank you for being there. You are a great nana!

My best friends in the world - Roberta, Charlee, Shanni, Kylie, Vix Bix, Julie,

Sarah L, Ruby, Laquois, Sarah T, Vetsky, Prue, Sandi, Danni, Jodie, Simone, PJ, Bedazzler, Beata, Rose, Deone, Tash, Rox, Debbie & Cam. You are the most wonderful, supportive, amazing friends and always in my big fat heart.

Ben – I love you so much. Thank you for all your help. You are my best friend, my love and my light. I couldn't have done his without you…

Oscar - Where do I start with you? (I'm crying already.) I cannot express the love I have for you. There are no words, just this feeling that consumes me. You are the light of my world, and I am so happy that you are part of my life.

You are my little man, my angel and my best friend. You are so cherished.

I love you always,

Mummy xxx

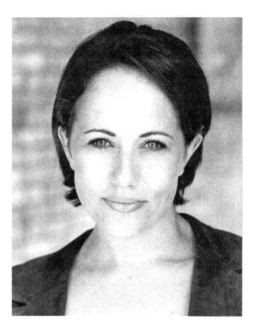

ABOUT THE AUTHOR

Kelly O'Brien was born in the small country town of McLaren Vale, South Australia. She began performing when she was 10 years old, and at 14 she was singing professionally.

Kelly soon developed her talents as a country artist and in 1990 she was crowned **South Australian Female Country Vocalist of the Year** and **Best new Talent** at the famous Australian Gympie Muster country festival a year later.

Kelly's first national television appearance was at the age of 18 on the talent show **New Faces** and soon she began regular TV spots on **Good Morning Australia, Carols in the Domain, Cartoon Network, Living with Style** and **Home and Away.** Kelly also beat 10,000 hopefuls to reach the final 12 in the second series of **Popstars** on Australian National Television.

Her commercial work has featured advertisements for 7-UP (directed by X-Men's Bryan Singer), **Mercedes Benz, H&M, Toyota, Nestlé** and Channel 4's **How to Look Good Naked.**

Kelly's musical theatre credits include Dinah in Andrew Lloyd Webber's **Starlight Express**, as well as lead roles in **Tropical nights, The Hunchback of Notre Dame, Spice Power** (the Australian Spice Girls tribute act), **Tonight's the Night** and **Hollywood in Concert.**

In 2004 Kelly secured a recording deal with Zyx music, re-releasing the hit single **Crucified** with the band **Glamrock.**

Kelly O'Brien now lives in London, working as a singer and comedienne. In early 2008 she launched a successful Dolly Parton tribute show.

Her greatest achievement to date (besides surviving childbirth) is the release of her first book **HELP! I can't see my foo foo…**

www.kellyobrien.co.uk

Printed in the United Kingdom
by Lightning Source UK Ltd.
134887UK00002B/70-114/P